The Keto Crockpot

Simple Delicious Ketogenic Crock Pot Recipes

To Help You Lose Weight Fast

TABLE OF CONTENTS

Introduction 7

   Why Keto? Why Crockpot? 7

   What to expect in this book 8

Chapter 1: What is the Ketogenic Diet? 9

Chapter 2: What Are the Benefits of the Ketogenic Diet? 11

   #1: You'll lose weight effortlessly 11

   #2: Your brainpower will explode!! 11

   #3: Your levels of endurance will exceed your expectations! 12

   #4: Goodbye hormonal imbalance! 12

   #5: You'll feel less hungry! Yay! 12

   #6: Your heart & cardiovascular system will get healthier 13

   #7: Your epilepsy symptoms could improve 13

   #8: You might finally manage to ease your migraines 13

   #9: You'll protect yourself against cancer 14

Chapter 3: Foods to Eat (and Enjoy!) & Foods to AVOID on the Keto Diet 15

   What You SHOULD Eat 16

   Meat & poultry 16

   Fish and seafood 16

   Eggs 16

   Full-fat dairy 16

   Fats, oils and delicious sauces 17

   Vegetables that grow above ground 17

   Herbs and spices 17

   Condiments 18

   Sweeteners 18

   Drinks 18

   Snacks 19

   Foods to Avoid 19

   Sugar 19

   Carbs & grains 20

   Beans & Lentils 20

   Margarine 21

   Alcohol, especially beer 21

   Fruit 21

   Unhealthy fats 22

Chapter 4: How to use the Keto diet to lose weight quickly 23

You can also expect: 23

How quickly can I lose weight? 23

How do I know if I'm in in ketosis? 24

Chapter 5: What to Do if You're *Not* Losing Weight on a Keto Diet 26

Tip #1: Eat fewer carbs 26

Tip #2: Include coconut oil 26

Tip #3: Check your protein intake 26

Tip #4: Stop cheating 26

Tip #5: Reduce your calories 27

Tip # 6: Be patient! 27

Tip #7: Avoid constant snacking and 'treats' 27

Tip #8: Stop weighing yourself so often 27

Tip #9: Avoid stress 28

Tip #10: Get enough sleep 28

Tip #11: Exercise *less* 28

Tip #12: Get some support 28

Tip #13: Avoid products with words like 'low carb', 'sugar-free' and 'fat free' 29

Tip #14: Drink more water and get enough electrolytes 29

Chapter 6: Keto FAQ 30

Apple 31

Low Carb Diet Tracker 31

Daily Carb- Nutrition Counter and Glucose Tracker 31

MyFitnessPal 31

Android 31

Low Carb Diet 31

My Fitness Pal 31

MyKeto 31

Chapter 6: Everything You Want to Know about Crockpots 34

What's a crock pot? 34

Why crockpots are great for Keto 34

What can you cook in a slow cooker? 35

Tip #1: Get prepared the night before 35

Tip #2: Go easy on the liquid 35

Tip #3: Go LOW 35

Tip #4: Leave it alone 35

Tip #5: Time it all to perfection 36

Chapter 7: Recipes 37
   Appetizers 37
      Italian Beef "Sandwiches" 37
      Spicy Stuffed Poblano Peppers 39
      Homemade Keto Meatloaf with Goat's Cheese and Spinach 40
      Buffalo Chicken Cream Cheese Fondue 41
      Garlicky Shrimp 42
      Sour Cream and Horseradish Cheese Dip 43
   Breakfast 44
      Ham, Ricotta and Spinach Breakfast Casserole 44
      Slow Cooker Spinach & Feta Quiche 45
      Keto Blueberry Breakfast Pancakes 46
      Keto Breakfast Brownies 47
      Spinach and Sausage Breakfast Frittata 48
      Jalapeño Popper Egg Cups 49
      Cinnamon Roll Oatmeal 50
      Maple Pecan Fat Bomb Bars 51
      Herby Bacon, Mozzarella and Mushroom Frittata 53
      Almond Crusted Keto Breakfast Quiche 54
      Chorizo-Cheese Breakfast Pie 55
      Keto Breakfast Cheese and Bacon Tacos 56
   Soups & Stews 57
      Ground Beef Minestrone Soup 57
      Thai Chicken Soup 58
      Lentil and Italian Sausage Soup 59
      Creamy Reuben Soup 60
      Spicy Jambalaya Soup 61
      Chicken and Kale Soup 62
      Cheesy Cauliflower Soup 63
      Rosemary, Turkey and Kale Soup 64
   Meat 65
      Lemongrass and Coconut Chicken Drumsticks 65
      Best Jerk Chicken in the WORLD! 66
      Mexican Crock Pot Fajita Chicken 67
      Slow Cooker Roasted Chicken with Lemon Parsley Butter 68
      Greek Chicken 69
      Sesame- Orange Chicken 70
      Italian Zucchini Meatloaf 71
      Chinese 5-Spice Pork Ribs 72

Pork Stew with Oyster Mushrooms 73

Chili Pulled Pork 74

Pork Chili Verde 75

New Mexico Carne Adovada 76

Slow Cooker Beef Stroganoff 77

Beef, Bacon & Cabbage Stew 78

Sweet Pepper Beef Tongue 79

Easy Slow Cooker Beef Chili 80

Coconut & Broccoli Chicken Curry 81

Easy Keto Ranch Chicken 82

Spiced Oxtail Stew 83

Chicken Pad Thai with Zucchini Noodles 84

Italian Hot Stuffed Peppers 86

Easy Korean Short Ribs 87

Deep Dish Cheese & Pepperoni Pizza with Cauliflower Crust 88

Seafood 89

Slow Cooker Trout with Orange and Pecans 89

Moqueca – Brazilian Fish Stew 90

Perfectly Poached Salmon 91

Shrimp Fra Diavolo 92

Keto Fish & Cheddar Pie 93

Dessert 95

Mocha Pudding Cake 95

Vanilla-Almond Keto Cheesecake 96

Almond & Raspberry Cream Cake 97

Fudgy Two-Layer Brownies 99

Lemon & Poppy Seed Cake 101

The Best Chocolate Cake You'll Taste All Year! 102

Extras 103

Cajun Seasoning 103

Avocado Cilantro Lime Sauce 104

Zucchini Tortillas 105

Final Words 106

Appendix: Conversion Tables 107

Introduction

Imagine if you could continue to enjoy rich, delicious foods that leave you feeling utterly spoilt and satisfied.

Imagine if you could wake up one morning and notice that you'd lost even more weight whilst you were sleeping...

Imagine if you didn't have to slave away for hours in the kitchen to prepare your food nor did you have had to compromise on your health to save time in the kitchen...

Sounds hard to believe, doesn't it? I'd go so far as to say *impossible.*

But you'll be amazed to hear that all of this is absolutely possible to enjoy a stress-free life and effortlessly lose weight in this way when you do two very important things.

You switch to a Ketogenic diet

You buy a crockpot (slow cooker) and start using it.

Doesn't sound very complicated at all, does it? So let me assure you that it's absolutely not. And most exciting of all, I'm here to tell you exactly how you can do it! Yay!

Why Keto? Why Crockpot?

The Ketogenic diet is one that is rapidly gaining popularity across the world with celebrities and health experts alike as a way of shifting weight and utterly transforming our lives so we can become the strongest, most vibrant versions of ourselves.

Because, as you probably know already, we're in a period of somewhat epidemic obesity which shows no sign of stalling. We try our luck with various slimming diets and other health fads, we spend thousands of dollars trying to get lean but despite our best efforts, nothing really seems to work.

This is how the Keto diet is much better.

Instead of filling us with fake low-fat foods that only make us sick and leaving us fatter than ever, it provides all the nutritious our body needs and tastes utterly amazing. You're not going to have to wave goodbye to butter, mayonnaise, avocados or any of this stuff and you will continue to lose weight.

What's even better is that you can make an incredible amount of Keto-friendly food right there in your crock pot. Just throw the ingredients into the pot, turn on the heat and walk away, only to return when your steaming, mouth-watering meal is ready. It really is a dream come true.

I've already written an in-depth book on the Ketogenic diet, so if you want to delve deeper and haven't yet read it, please do download it here. That first book was incredibly popular and since it was published and as a result I've had a ton of requests for a crockpot cookbook. So, I've decided to create it for you here- I hope you really enjoy it!

A few notes before we get started- I've tried to avoid using jargon and other technical terms so even the absolute beginner can start benefiting from this transformative diet in the easiest way possible.

What to expect in this book

I'll kick off by explaining what the Ketogenic diet is and how it can benefit your life (you won't only lose weight, but transform your overall health too.) Then we'll take a look at which foods you can continue to enjoy and which ones you need to start avoiding, and why. Then we'll move on to discussing how you can use the Ketogenic specifically to lose weight, and I'll help you out with some troubleshooting and answer your FAQS.

Then we'll round it all up with a quick look at what a crockpot is and what it can do to make your life a ton easier, then we'll dive right into the recipe section. Here you'll find more than 60 recipes ranging from breakfasts, starters, desserts, mains and much more (plus a few bonus Keto-friendly side-dishes at the end.

So, let's not sit around here talking- let's get exploring the love affair between the Ketogenic diet, your crockpot and weight loss!

Chapter 1: What is the Ketogenic Diet?

If you've read my previous book *"Ketogenic Diet 101- The Complete Beginner's Guide to Eating Keto"*, you'll know that the Keto diet is the perfect way to indulge in all those thick, delicious sauces, creamy butter and soft mayonnaise without having to worry about your waistline.

In fact, it will help you lose weight almost effortlessly whilst still enjoying every single bit of food you eat, without having to eat rabbit food and whilst still enjoying the finder things in life.

Like the Atkins diet or the LCHF diet, it's very low carb, but unlike Atkins (which emphasizes lots of protein), the Ketogenic diet is low in protein. This is because your body is a very clever thing and can convert protein into carbs when it needs to. Carbs are the very thing we're trying to avoid.

As you might know, carbs are essential to fuel your body and your brain but that's not the only option when it comes to nutrition. You see, your body is amazing and can adapt switch its main fuel source from carbs to fat.

If you're barely eating any carbs this means your body will make that switch and the weight will quite literally drop off you! I've woken up in the morning to find myself skinnier than the night before- I was astonished!

I prefer to keep science and numbers out of it so I can keep it simple for you, but know that you'll be eating a diet of around 70-80% fat, around 25% protein and 5% carbs.

The transitions from using carbs as a main energy course to fats doesn't happen overnight- you can expect to experience the following three stages:

You start eating a high fat low carb diet.

Your body starts to adjust to using fat as fuel instead of carbs, and you might notice a few 'detox' symptoms which can last anywhere from two to seven days.

Eventually, your body enters a state called '**Ketosis**' where your body now runs on fats alone.

How does ketosis work?

In the beginning when you first make the switch to a fat-based diet, you might not notice much difference because your liver contains a store of glucose which will keep you going for a while. Once this runs out, and there aren't sufficient carbs in your diet, your body starts converting the fat in your diet to something called ketones which is a fuel which works more efficiently than carbs. This is ketosis.

If you're not getting enough calories from your diet, your body will start searching for alternative forms of fat and will discover any excess fat hanging around your body, including that belly fat, your love handles, your thighs, your butt, your arm 'wobble' and much more.

The result of all of this is lasting, amazing weight loss.

Is the Keto diet suitable for everyone?

The Keto diet is suitable for most adults of all ages, and some children too (but only under the supervision of a doctor.) However, there are some groups of people who need to be extra cautious before they make these kinds of major dietary changes.

They include:

Diabetics and those on insulin medication

People with high blood pressure

Pregnancy or breastfeeding women

Generally speaking, it's *always* a good idea to visit your doctor before you make any kind of diet or exercise changes so do the sensible thing and make an appointment with your physician first.

Feeling clued up? That's great! But did you know that the Ketogenic diet isn't just great for people like you and I who want to lose weight and feel incredible. It also has some great therapeutic benefits. Turn the page and find out more!

Chapter 2: What Are the Benefits of the Ketogenic Diet?

Chances are that you haven't just downloaded this book at random, hoping that it will be interesting and give you some more food ideas (at least I hope not!!) You're hoping that the Ketogenic can benefit your lifestyle, your body and your health.

You want the same incredible weight-loss that you've seen so many celebrities and fitness experts RAVE about, and you want to get that effortless beach-ready body that you've heard so much about.

But as I just mentioned at the end of the last chapter, the Keto diet isn't just about losing weight the fun way. It will also benefit your health in so many ways so you can become the strongest, and healthiest version of yourself you could ever imagine.

So, before we hop onwards towards the recipes, let's take a few moments to look at all the benefits that the Keto diet can have. Are you ready? Let's take a look!

#1: You'll lose weight effortlessly

Yep, as we know, the Keto diet is brilliant for losing excess weight and allowing the slimmer, vibrant you to emerge from the shell. You'll shift weight whilst you sleep as your body burns that belly fat away until you look leaner, fitter and ready for anything!

#2: Your brainpower will explode!!

Don't get worried- your brains aren't about to leap from your skull and make a nasty mess over the kitchen. What I mean is that you'll discover just how mentally agile, creative and intelligent you can be. You'll learn brand new things even more easily than before, that brain fog will disappear and it will feel like ANYTHING is possible.

This comes down to the fact that dietary fats have a nourishing and protective effect on the nervous system which flicks your brain power to turbo and helps you become unstoppable.

#3: Your levels of endurance will exceed your expectations!

Have you ever noticed how you go for a run or take part in another sports activity, and despite a great start, there comes a time when you run out of energy and 'hit the wall'? This is because you've run out of glucose to fuel your body, in much as the same way as running out of gas in your car.

Here's where Keto is different. Because instead of using stored glucose (which has its limits), your entire body will be running on fat which will keep you going for a very, very long time.

Hello ultra-endurance race!

(Note: if you are following a Keto diet as an aid to your endurance training, please give your body at least two weeks to adjust and monitor your electrolytes and fluids very closely.)

#4: Goodbye hormonal imbalance!

Global levels of hormone-related imbalances are now at epidemic levels. This includes insulin-sensitivity, type 2 diabetes, metabolic syndrome, PMT, PCOS, adrenal fatigue and many others. The reason? The Western diet.

The Keto diet is the perfect remedy. Because unlike the western diet which is packed full of carbs, sugars and other substances which disrupt your overall hormone balance, the Keto diet actually helps keep your hormones healthy.

The fats and cholesterol in the Keto diet help produce and regulate your natural hormone production, rebalancing your hormone levels, easing your hormonal symptoms and helping you feel human again.

It also reduces your risk of developing diabetes and improves your body's ability to respond to any sugars it eventually encounters. Awesome!

#5: You'll feel less hungry! Yay!

There's one major problem with the regular kind of slimming diets- they just leave you feeling deprived, hungry and desperate to stuff your face with whatever 'banned' food there is. You see, these foods usually lack the essential fats which signal to your body that you've eaten enough and switch those hunger hormones off.

This is where the Keto diet really shines! As you know, the Keto diet is really high in those fats so you'll stay satisfied and keep away from the cookie tin. Additionally, scientists believe that these fats might also play an interesting role in switching on and off your hunger hormones, ghrelin and leptin. Watch this space for more details!

#6: Your heart & cardiovascular system will get healthier

Most people think that fats are the very thing responsible for heart disease, high blood cholesterol levels and other associated problems. And it's not their fault. After all, we've been told for decades now that this is the problem. However, scientists are now doing an about-turn and admitting that they got it all wrong- it's actually the carbs and sugars that are doing the damage. (Eeek!)

But don't worry. By following the Keto diet, you'll be reducing levels of those dangerous triglycerides in your blood, raising the amount of GOOD cholesterol in your blood (HDL) and protecting your body from heart disease and associated illness. Now if that's not a great reason alone to eat more butter, I don't know what is!

#7: Your epilepsy symptoms could improve

Doctors first explored the Ketogenic as a way of easing symptoms of epilepsy for children who were unresponsive to medication but needed help. It was highly successful and allowed many epileptic children to go completely med-free for the first time in their lives.

It could benefit you too if you suffer from epilepsy. However, please contact your doctor if you are interested in exploring this- the diet needs to be closely monitored in this context.

#8: You might finally manage to ease your migraines

Let's be honest- migraines are a pain in the b***. There's nothing worse than looking forward to a great night out with friends, hanging with your partner or chilling with the kids. Then along comes a migraine and your only option is to lock yourself away in a darkened room and roll around in agony...It's definitely *not* my favorite way to spend a weekend.

Thankfully, the Ketogenic diet could help. Scientists are still investigating the full benefits of the diet for migraines, but signs point to the fact that the Keto diet reduces levels of glutamate in the brain which has been linked to attacks.

Here's a link to a really interesting article on this matter.

#9: You'll protect yourself against cancer

Ever wondered why there are so many cases of cancer around these days and victims are becoming younger and younger? If so, you're not the only one- so many of my friends have lost their lives to this unforgiving disease.

Scientists have discovered that carbs, especially *sugars* feed cancerous cells and could increase your chances of falling victim too. This means that following a Keto diet could potential reduce your risk of suffering from cancer, and could help in its treatment. In fact, many people claim that Keto has cured them of cancer. Certainly something for us to think about.

However, please don't presume that I mean that you should do the same. I'm not a medical doctor and I would never advise that you follow my advice without consulted a qualified practitioner first. Having said that, it's certainly worth mentioning to your oncologist.

Surprised? I thought you might be. Because it usually the slimming benefits that get covered a whole lot in the press but the other wider benefits often get forgotten.

We could also add great energy and lust for life to the list, plus the fact that Keto helps you sleep better, feel better and start cooking real food from scratch. You could say it has benefits in all areas of your life!

Hopefully, you're really sold on the benefits of the Ketogenic diet and you're ready to watch the weight simply fall off, see your health improve and start feeling in the best shape of your life. So, you're probably eager to know what kinds of foods you can enjoy (and if you really can eat a ton of fats!!) and which foods you'll need to avoid. Turn to the next chapter and I'll explain all!

Chapter 3: Foods to Eat (and Enjoy!) & Foods to AVOID on the Keto Diet

From reading all the info I've shared so far about the Keto diet, you might be feeling slightly apprehensive and unsure of what *exactly* you can eat. You've probably got a ton of questions floating around in your head, such as;

"Will I have to quit bread? Are sweet treats completely off the menu? Will I have to eat dull, unappetizing foods? What about socializing?"

So, let me put your mind at ease and reassure you that the Keto diet isn't as boring as you might be thinking.

In fact, I'd go so far as to say **that the Keto diet is perfect if you love your food and you're not willing to compromise on taste** for the sake of losing a few (or many) pounds or staying healthy. Sound good?

Now I'm about to give you some long lists of the foods you can eat and enjoy and let you know which foods you need to avoid on the Keto diet, but don't feel overwhelmed. You see, the Keto diet *isn't* as difficult as you think. You simply need to bear the following in mind:

Eat healthy fats. Eat meat, fish, poultry and seafood. Eat some veggies. Avoid carbs.

So, without any further ado, here are the lists. Enjoy!

What You SHOULD Eat

Meat & poultry

Eat any meat you like, including:

Beef

Pork

Lamb

Game

Chicken

Turkey

Organ meats

Choose organic or grass-fed as much as possible and don't be afraid to eat the fat- it's good for you.

Fish and seafood

Everything is great! Include:

Fatty fish such as salmon, mackerel, sardines or herring to keep your omega 3 levels up and keep your nervous system healthy

White fish like cod

(However, make sure you avoid <u>breaded</u> fish!)

Eggs

Eat any kind of eggs you like as they're a great source of protein on a Keto diet.

You can serve them any way you like, including boiled, fried, scrambled, in an omelet, cooked into 'breads' or any other way you can find. Choose free-range and organic whenever you can.

Full-fat dairy

You can eat any kind of dairy product you like, as long as it's not low-fat or zero fat. This includes butter, cream, sour cream, Greek or Turkish yoghurt and high fat cheeses.

However, avoid drinking large quantities of milk- the carbs in milk really add up after a while.

Fats, oils and delicious sauces

Yum! You can eat plenty of oils, fats and rich sauces on the Keto diet. You can include:
Butter
Cream
Coconut oil
Olive oil
Ghee
Chicken fat
Avocados
Mayonnaise
High-fat sauces

Vegetables that grow above ground

Whilst vegetables do contain carbs, not all are built the same. You can still enjoy low carb veggies such as:
Cauliflower
Broccoli
Cabbage
Brussels sprouts
Green leafy veggies like kale, collards, bok choy & spinach,
Asparagus
Zucchini
Eggplant
Olives
Mushrooms
Cucumber
Lettuce
Avocado
Onions and garlic

Herbs and spices

There are absolutely no restrictions when it comes to herbs and spices- you can really indulge and bring plenty of flavor to your meals. These include blended seasonings like Mexican, Indian and Lemon-pepper and individual spices like cumin, cilantro and sesame seeds. Make sure any store-bought blends are sugar-free and gluten-free.

You can also add plenty of fresh herbs like cilantro, parsley, chives, basil and so on. Why not grow your own on a windowsill so you can enjoy them whenever the urge takes you!

Condiments

You will need to avoid some sauces on the Keto diet as they contain high levels of sugars and carbs (ketchup and BBQ are off the menu, I'm afraid.) But don't worry- there are still loads you can enjoy guilt-free. They include the following:

Soy Sauce

Lemon and lime juice

Sriracha Sauce

Homemade mayonnaise

Mustards – Dijon and Stone-ground versions

Hot sauces (check they're sugar-free)

Salad dressings (if homemade)

Sweeteners

Sweeteners are a tricky issue on the Keto diet. Purists generally like to avoid them altogether because for some people, they increase cravings for sugar and carbs. However, if you want to make yourself some sweet, healthy treats, they are the perfect alternative to regular sugar. Choose between:

Erythritol

Stevia

Splenda (I don't use this, personally, but many do)

Brand-name sugar replacements

Drinks

You can enjoy plenty of different drinks on the Keto diet, provided you keep it nice and simple.

Opt for the following:

Water

Coffee (especially with cream or served Bulletproof Coffee style)

Tea

Yes, you *can* also enjoy some alcohol drinks on the Keto diet, but you do have to be careful which ones you select as some are pretty high in carbs.

If you do want something alcoholic, why not indulge in a glass of champagne, red wine or white wine instead? Whilst they *do* contain some carbs, the levels are relatively small- just 1-2g per beverage. Also suitable are whisky, tequila, Vodka and soda, Dry Martini or Brandy which all contain zero carbs.

Snacks

Life wouldn't be living if it weren't for the occasional snack to see you through the day. The trouble is, it's not always easy to find low-carb options. The following are all my own go-to snack ideas:

Hard-boiled eggs
Crispy bacon rashers
Ham filled with cucumber & avocado and rolled up.
2-3 celery sticks with nut butter
Fermented foods like sauerkraut and Kimchi
Pork rinds or cracklings
Nuts and seeds (avoid cashew nuts)
Fat Bombs (see my Beginner's Guide to Keto book for recipes)

Foods to Avoid

I always like to start with the positive bit- the foods you can eat and enjoy, but now, it's time for the rest- what you need to keep out of your diet. Shall we take a look?

Sugar

Carbs and sugar are much the same thing- if you need to limit one, the same will apply for the others. However, don't think that skipping the added sugar in your coffee, avoiding candy bars and skipping soda is all you need to do. Many processed foods also contain sugar as does fruit.

Generally speaking, it's best to avoid all of these if you're serious about following the Ketogenic diet.

Soft drinks
Fruit yoghurts
Premade cereal bars
Smoothies
Candy
Juice
Sports drinks
Chocolate
Cake
Buns
Pastries
Ice cream
Donuts
Cookies
Breakfast cereals

Carbs & grains

The following foods are also high carb. Avoid them all!

Wheat

Barley

Oats

Rice

Rye

Corn

Quinoa

Millet

Sorghum

Bulgur

Amaranth

Sprouted grains

Buckwheat

So obviously, you'll also have to avoid these foods (as they contain the above ingredients):

Bread

Pasta

Rice

Potatoes

French fries

Potato chips

Porridge

Oats

Muesli

It's important to mention that you should also avoid wholegrain products as they are just as bad as the processed version as they are packed full of carbs.

Beans & Lentils

Beans and lentils are very high carb, so avoid them all...

Kidney beans

Chickpeas

Black beans

Lentils

Green peas

Lima beans

Pinto beans
White beans
Fava beans

Margarine

Let's be honest- margarine isn't really a food. It's more a food-like product, devoid of any nutritional benefit (apart from those chemical additives) and containing a whole host of nasty side effects.

Turn to those healthy fats instead.

Alcohol, especially beer

Most alcoholic drinks are so high carb, you may as well consider them to be like a bag of candy or a loaf of bread. That's not even mentioning those drinks high in sugars like cocktails and other alcoholic soda drinks. Avoid them all.

However, check out the section on drinks in the 'foods you can eat' section for some great alcoholic and non-alcoholic alternatives.

Fruit

Sorry if you're a bit fruit lover- you'll need to steer clear of fruit as much as possible on the Keto diet. You see, Keto avoids all sugars, including natural sugars found in fruit.

This includes fruit juice, dried fruit and fruit smoothies, unless they're Keto friendly. Having said that, small amounts of low carb fruit such as berries are fine (very) occasionally.

Fruits to avoid include:

Bananas
Pineapples
Papaya
Apples
Oranges
Grapes
Mangos
Tangerines
All fruit juices
Fruit smoothies
Dried fruits like raisins, dates, dried mango, etc.
Fruit syrups
Fruit concentrates

Unhealthy fats

Not all fats are made the same way- there are some oils that can be quite harmful to your health and should be avoided. These are highly processed and contain carcinogenic properties.

These include:

Soybean oil
Canola oil
Corn oil
Grapeseed oil
Peanut oil
Sesame oil
Sunflower oil

So, there you are! A list of all the foods you can eat and those you should avoid. I've kept it nice and simple for you- simply remember the basics and try to stick with no-carb, unprocessed foods as much as possible.

Before we get on with the recipes, I'd like to dedicate some time to explaining more about how you can use the Keto diet to aid weight-loss, and I'll also share some great tips that will help you get over those stumbling blocks and discover the healthiest, slimmest version of yourself ever.

Chapter 4: How to use the Keto diet to lose weight quickly

As you've seen already, the very core of Keto is astonishing weight loss, incredible improvements in health and wellness *and* protection against all kinds of illnesses.

So why is Keto so beneficial for weight loss? How can you get maximum benefits in your own life and fit into your favorite jeans again? And what do you do when it doesn't seem to work? Let me help...

The Ketogenic diet is better than other diets

Keto is *much* superior to other weight loss programs you might have tried in the past because of the diet's ability to shear weight off all your problem areas without you doing very much at all apart from enjoying great food and taking care of yourself.

Additionally, Keto does away with those horrible cravings you often get on a slimming diet and helps you to feel satisfied, energized and glowing with health. You won't get those sugar highs and lows so you'll stick to your diet more effortlessly and feel great as you do so.

You can also expect:

Long term weight loss
Lower blood pressure
Reduced cholesterol
Fewer cravings
Better insulin resistance
Less inflammation
Lean, healthy weight loss (not just staying puffy but getting smaller)

How quickly can I lose weight?

The answer to this question really depends on your body type, your activity levels, your usual diet and what you're eating on the Ketogenic diet. You'll first have to enter through that period of Ketosis (where your body switches to using fat as its supply) before you lose any weight at all.

If you want to speed things up, make sure you keep your carb intake very low (below 20g for best results), make sure you're drinking enough water and getting adequate rest and also exercise on an empty stomach.

How do I know if I'm in in ketosis?

If you listen to your body, you'll usually know when ketosis is happening. Watch for tell-tale signs like:

A fruity or metallic taste in your mouth or your breath smelling like old-fashioned pear drops

Short-term weakness (in the early days)

Short-term decrease in physical performance (in the early days)

Weight loss caused by fat or water loss

Digestive issues

Reduced appetite

Increased energy (in the later stages)

Better focus and concentration

Better sleep

When you are in ketosis, your body will release ketones in your urine which you can test with special sticks easily available at any pharmacy. Be aware that they're not the most reliable of tests. You can also use something called a blood ketone meter which is more accurate but more expensive.

However, in my opinion you don't need either of these things- simply monitoring your body and watching for changes will be enough.

A few words on Keto flu

Keto flue is a period of 'detox' where your body adjusts to getting its fuel from fats instead of carbs. This can often feel like a period of withdrawal, like the detox feeling you experience if you've ever given up caffeine or cigarettes.

For some the transition can be easy and over quickly but other can find it more difficult and experience symptoms such as:

Headaches

Sickness

Stomach ache/ diarrhea

Foggy thinking

Sleepiness

This is completely normal and will be over within a few days to a week. It's also very much worth it when you consider the incredible benefits that come at the end!

The following will help you get through this period:
Drink lots of water
Get enough electrolytes
Eat enough fat
Go easy on the protein (so your body doesn't immediately turn them to carbs)
Rest!

Remember, the amount of weight loss you experience and how quickly it happens comes down to YOU can how strictly you are following the Keto diet. However, sometimes it doesn't happen as quickly as we'd like.

So, what do we do? How do we keep losing weight when we've reached a plateau? Turn to the next chapter and I'll trouble-shoot your issues!

Chapter 5: What to Do if You're *Not* Losing Weight on a Keto Diet

You're doing all the right things; you're following the diet, you've vastly reduced your carb intake and you're even getting plenty of exercise to help you shift weight.

But, horror of horrors! You're still not losing weight. Or perhaps you were at the beginning when you first went Keto but not you've stalled a little and aren't sure how to get rid of that remaining body fat.

Don't worry- I've got your back! There are all common things to happen when you're using the Keto diet for weight loss and there are lots of things we can do to help you get on track. Here are my top tips.

Tip #1: Eat fewer carbs

It's surprising how many grams of carb are there hidden in your food, even if you think you're doing pretty well and if you don't take control of them, they can really interfere with your weight loss. So, it's time to slash them.

Tip #2: Include coconut oil

Coconut oil is a wonderful fat which is easily digestible and contains fats called medium-chain triglycerides (MCTs for short). These are less likely to be stored by your body as fat, are easily converted into ketones and help you enter ketosis.

Tip #3: Check your protein intake

Protein can be a tricky issue on Keto as too much will disrupt ketosis (because it will be converted into glycogen in your liver) and too little will leave you feeling hungry and more likely to overeat. However, if you're eating a regular diet this shouldn't be a problem. It's those protein supplements that you might want to avoid.

Tip #4: Stop cheating

Sure, you might think that a tiny nibble of some chocolate or a little tiny crust of bread won't make a difference overall but you'd be amazed. Because all it takes is a tiny bit of carbs and your body will swing right out of ketosis and you'll be back to square one. I'm not going to tell you that you can't eat these things, but ask yourself, *is it really worth it?*

Tip #5: Reduce your calories

Whilst we can eat fats on the Keto diet, that doesn't mean you don't ever have to think about calories. You can still get fat on Keto. Yes, that's right. At the end of the day, if you're fueling your engine with more gas than it needs, the excess is going to have to go somewhere, right? Watch your calories and make sure you're keeping your fat intake between 60-75% of your daily calories.

Tip # 6: Be patient!

Don't expect that you'll see results overnight because, like other slimming diets, it does take time to see results. So be patient, give it some time and you'll soon notice how much looser your jeans are becoming, or how much slimming your face is looking! Awesome!

Likewise, if you're almost at your goal weight, you can expect to see the weight loss slowing down. This is completely normal and nothing to worry about. Just keep on doing what you're doing!

Tip #7: Avoid constant snacking and 'treats'

The occasional low-carb snack, treat or desert is absolutely fine and won't do your diet too much hard. But if you start indulging in them on a regular basis (especially baked foods containing stevia or erythritol), you increase your chances of struggling with food cravings and overeating. I've included several yummy treats in the recipe section for you, but please enjoy them occasionally. Stick to real foods the rest of the time.

Also make sure you're not overdoing snacking on dairy or the nuts as these do contain some carbs and could throw your body out ketosis, as well as being quite high calorie and hard to resist once you get going! If you really must snack, stick to low carb veg like broccoli, cauliflower, zucchini, and cucumber instead.

Tip #8: Stop weighing yourself so often

Your weight will naturally fluctuate throughout the day, and if you're female, throughout the month too which might cause you to panic when there really is no need. These increases and decreases are usually down to water retention or hormones and don't mean that your diet is failing. Either don't weigh yourself at all or stick to just weighing yourself once per week. A great way to track your weight loss is to use a measuring tape or check the fit of your clothes instead.

Tip #9: Avoid stress

When you are stressed, your body produces a hormonal called cortisol which affects your overall hormone balance, disrupts your blood sugar levels, causes cravings of sweet foods and caffeine and also causes you to store more weight around your stomach area. This is exactly what we don't want.

So, if you have a stressful life or you feel overwhelmed, sad or lonely, please take steps to address this. It's not a sign of weakness- you just need support. Remember, stress isn't just physical but can be psychological or emotional too.

Find ways you can reduce the stress in your life such as learning breathing exercises, taking long walks, doing the things you love, learning how to meditate, practicing martial arts or yoga or treat yourself to a holiday!

Tip #10: Get enough sleep

If you're not sleeping enough, your body can't produce the right hormones to signal when you're hungry or you're full and also it will have a hard time regulating your blood sugar levels and helping you feel well. So, do your body a favor and get at least 7-9 hours of sleep per night. It's vital for your health and your weight-loss.

Tip #11: Exercise *less*

Yes, you really did read that right. If you're struggling to lose weight, you should start exercising much less than you. Over-exercise can actually do more harm than good as it increases your appetite quite significantly and can stress the body (see above.) Stick to three x 30-minute sessions per week.

Tip #12: Get some support

It's much easier to stick to a Keto diet when you have a great support network around you. They'll be there to feed you with extra information, support you if you're struggling with an issue in your life and also help you have that sense of team spirit which can help you stick to your plan. Head to Facebook and look up the Ketogenic diet in the groups there- you'll find plenty of help.

Tip #13: Avoid products with words like 'low carb', 'sugar-free' and 'fat free'

These products contain lots of horrible additives which are terrible for your body, in additional to artificial sweeteners which can also cause insulin spikes and damage your body, as well as jeopardizing your weight loss efforts. Again, stick with real food.

Tip #14: Drink more water and get enough electrolytes

Water helps to metabolize your body fat, keeps your body working efficiently and also helps to reduce your appetite so make sure you're drinking plenty. Also ensure you're getting enough electrolytes such as magnesium, potassium and sodium for optimal health. A multivitamin and mineral could be a good idea.

These tips have worked wonders with several of my friends who have turned to me for advice when they encountered problems losing weight on the Keto diet. And let me assure you that their stories had a happy ending- they all reached their ideal weight and are healthy, happy, vibrant, and still following a Keto plan.

Of course, I was always there to help them out when they most needed it, answering their questions and providing the support whenever necessary to help them achieve their dreams and goals. And although I can't be right there with you (*I wish I could!*), I certainly can help you out a ton by addressing the questions before you even ask them!

Turn to the following chapter and have a read through my FAQs before we get started.

Chapter 6: Keto FAQ

In case I've missed anything so far in this book, I've gathered together some answers to the questions I get asked most often. Here they are:

Should I be taking a supplement?

Everybody, no matter what diet they are following, should be taking a daily multivitamin and mineral supplement to ensure they're getting everything their body needs. In an ideal world, we'd all be getting absolutely everything we need from our food, but it just doesn't work like that these days. I'd recommend the following:

Multivitamin and mineral
Magnesium
Vitamin B-complex
Vitamin D (or make sure you're getting plenty of sunshine)
Potassium

Remember- I'm not a doctor so please do check with a medical professional before taking any of these supplements.

Do I have to measure my carb intake?

It's really up to you and how strictly you want to adhere to the Keto diet. Provided you're eating the right amounts of fat and protein and avoiding carbs as much as possible, you should be fine. If you want to get serious or you're using the Keto diet to help treat a medical condition or for endurance sports, then this might be worth doing.

The easiest way is through an app you can download to your cell phone, such as one of these:

Apple

Low Carb Diet Tracker

https://itunes.apple.com/us/app/low-carb-diet-tracker-pro-by-carb-manager/id410089731?mt=8

Daily Carb- Nutrition Counter and Glucose Tracker

https://itunes.apple.com/us/app/daily-carb-nutrition-counter-and-glucose-tracker/id536425111?mt=8

MyFitnessPal https://itunes.apple.com/us/app/calorie-counter-diet-tracker-by-myfitnesspal/id341232718?mt=8

Android

Low Carb Diet

https://play.google.com/store/apps/details?id=com.deluxapps.carb.foods.guide&hl=en

My Fitness Pal

https://play.google.com/store/apps/details?id=com.myfitnesspal.android&hl=en

MyKeto

https://play.google.com/store/apps/details?id=com.prestigeworldwide.keto&hl=en

I haven't personally tried any of these so give them a go and let me know what you think!

I'm constipated! What can I do?
As your body transitions to a Keto diet, it's going to be making some major internal adjustments. That means you might suffer from the odd bout of constipation or other digestive changes along the way. But fear not! There are plenty of things you can do about this:

Take a tablespoon of olive oil or coconut oil
Drink lots of water
Eat more vegetables (the low-carb kind!)
Drink tea or coffee (Bulletproof coffee is a great remedy- see the recipe here)

Eat chia seeds or flax seeds

How about alcohol?

Alcohol is a tricky one because it tends to be very high carb- especially drinks like beer, cocktails and sweetened syrup-based spirits. I'd advise that you stay away from alcohol as much as you can. Of course, that doesn't mean you can't treat yourself to the occasional glass of wine or glass of clear liquor. I've written more about this in the foods you can eat section. Go and check it out if you want more info.

Can vegetarians follow Keto?

The good news is...yes you can. The bad news is...it's going to be very difficult for you at times.

Let's start with the good news! The Keto diet is based on fats, with low levels of protein and minimal carbs, but that's not to say that these fats (or protein, for that matter) need to come from animal sources. In fact, I have several vegetarian friends who say they have no trouble at all sticking to Keto *and* vegetarianism. Fats are easy on a vegetarian diet- simply add some extra avocados, butter, oils, cheese and eggs and you'll easily tick the box.

The rest of the vegetarian diet can be quite problematic though. You see, most vegetarians tend to rely on beans and lentils as their main source of protein which is something you can't do on Keto. My friend eats plenty of eggs and cheese for protein, topped up with low-carb nuts and seeds and does just fine on it.

Another problem is going to be the veggies and fruit. Both of these food groups tend to be very high carb, so they are going to have to be largely off the menu. Instead you should eat low carb varieties like cucumber, lettuce, spinach, zucchini and cabbage instead.

Be aware that your weight-loss will be slower on the vegetarian keto diet than it would be otherwise.

Isn't eating all that fat bad for your health?

No! The Keto diet emphasizes eating healthy dietary fats instead of those harmful vegetable oils that are packed into the average western diet.

However, I understand your worries because for such a long time we were told that saturated fats were bad and vegetable fats were good. We were told there was a link between cholesterol, saturated fat consumption and heart disease, but now we know that this just isn't true. Stick with those healthy dietary fats and you'll be fine.

Can I work out on the Keto diet?

The Keto diet has been proven to be an excellent diet for those who are interested in endurance sports like running, marathons and long-distance races as well as people who lift weight and play other sports, so that answer is YES!

If you run, play sports or do aerobics, you can just stick to regular Keto. But if you lift weights, you might want to take a more tailored approach. You see, carbohydrates have shown to be better than fat at building muscles and aiding recovery post workout- you might want to tailor your Keto diet accordingly.

There are two ways people often do this- by using a Targeted Ketogenic Diet and the Cyclical Ketogenic Diet. The first allows you to eat the ideal amount of carbs for your workout and then return to ketosis, and the other allows to cycle through period of Keto and a carb-rich diet. If you plan on doing either of these, please seek further advice from a trained professional.

Chapter 6: Everything You Want to Know about Crockpots

This isn't just your average Keto book, is it? It's also a book about cooking delicious, mouth-watering foods in your slow cooker which nourish your body and indulge your taste buds.

However, you might not have used one before, nor understand what they're all about, so let me give you a quick rundown.

What's a crock pot?

A crock pot (or slow cooker) is an electrical device that you can place on your counter, plug in and start cooking. Using an internal heating element, the food cooks at a low temperature over a period of several hours so you can prepare your next meal and simply walk away, letting technology do most of the hard work for you. Awesome, don't you think?

Almost all slow cookers have a variety of settings including high, medium, low or keep warm which you can use to adjust the time you want to take to cook your food. For example, in many of the recipes in this book, you'll hear me say *'cook on high for 3-4 hours or low for 7-8'*.

Some of the most basic models need to be switched on and off manually, but many newer models also come with a computerized timer facility that you can use to delay the start of cooking, or control the cooking without you ever having to be there.

Why crockpots are great for Keto

If I'm completely honest, I'd have to admit that crockpots are the best thing ever invented when it comes to helping you live a healthy life with the minimum of effort.

Because thanks to these brilliant kitchen appliances, you *don't* have to spend hours slaving away in the kitchen to eat healthily. In most cases, you can just throw everything in the pot, switch on, walk away and return after a few hours to find an incredible meal waiting for you.

What can you cook in a slow cooker?

Great question! You can cook pretty much anything in a slow cooker, provided it needs heat! That includes foods like roast chicken, deliciously fragrant and spicy curries, stews, soups, indulgence chocolate cakes, tender pork ribs and much more. Turn to the recipe section to find out more!

A few tips on using a crock pot

Here are a few tips to create incredible food in your crockpot.

Tip #1: Get prepared the night before

If you're choosing to cook your evening meal whilst you're out at work, get organized the night before. Simply prepare your ingredients and pop them into your slow cooker then place the whole thing in the fridge overnight. Then all you need to do in the morning is pull it out, turn it on and start cooking. Awesome!

Tip #2: Go easy on the liquid

As slow cookers retain moisture, it's a good idea not to go overboard with the liquid, even if you think you might need a bit more. Unlike cooking on the stove, excess water doesn't evaporate so will stick around inside the slow cooker, adding to the flavor and making everything wonderfully moist it simply melts in your mouth. Mmmm....

Tip #3: Go LOW

If you really care about flavors, try to use the low setting most often. Not only will this save on electricity, it will also bring out the flavors in your food, which is extra brilliant when you're cooking delicious cuts of meat or fish.

Tip #4: Leave it alone

Don't be tempted to keep peeping at your food or stirring when you really don't have to. You'll only let that valuable steam escape and ruin your lovely meal inside.

Tip #5: Time it all to perfection

All the recipes in this book have cooking times provided, but I'm assuming that you're not planning to stick with these and you'll actually want to get creative with your own recipes. Here's a great guide that will help you work out how long to cook new dishes for in your slow cooker:

Regular time	Time in a slow cooker
15 - 30 mins	1 - 2 hours on High, or 4 - 6 hours on Low
30 mins - 1 hour	2 - 3 hours on High or 5 - 7 hours on Low
1 - 2 hours	3 - 4 hours on High or 6 - 8 hours on Low
2 - 4 hours	4 - 6 hours on High or 8 - 12 hours on Low

So now we've got all that out of the way, are you ready for your recipes? I thought so. Let's go!

Chapter 7: Recipes

Appetizers
Italian Beef "Sandwiches"

Let's kick of this book with a really exciting recipe that you probably aren't expecting-these Italian Beef 'Sandwiches'. With all the herby flavor of your regular Italian favorites and topped with a delicious melted cheese lid, you'll be proud to present these at your next dinner party, Enjoy!

Serves: 6
Time: 7-8 hours

Ingredients
- 2 ½ lbs. (1.1kg) beef
- 2 tablespoons butter or lard
- 1 teaspoon dried basil
- 1 teaspoon dried oregano
- 1 teaspoon dried crushed rosemary
- 1 teaspoon garlic powder
- 1 teaspoon onion powder
- Salt and pepper to taste
- 1/2 cup (120ml) water
- 1 tablespoon red wine vinegar
- 2 tablespoon Dijon mustard
- 6 large Portobello mushroom caps
- Shredded mozzarella, to taste

Method
1. Start by heating the butter or lard in your slow cooker over a high heat.
2. Meanwhile, throw all the spices into a bowl and mix them together.
3. Throw the beef into the bowl and rub the spices in with your hands.
4. Now take your beef into the slow cooker and cook on each side for approx. 5 minutes.
5. Add the water and the vinegar then cook on low for 7-8 hours.

6. Remove the beef from the slow cooker and shred well.
7. Add the Dijon mustard into the liquids still in the slow cooker and stir well to combine then return the beef to the pot and stir well to combine.
8. Meanwhile, roast the Portobello mushrooms in the oven with salt, pepper and a dash of oil for around 10 minutes then place onto a plate.
9. Top with shredded beef and top with the shredded mozzarella.
10. Serve and enjoy!

Spicy Stuffed Poblano Peppers

If you're a fan of spicy comfort foods, you're going to adore these stuffed peppers. With a tiny amount of net carbs and packed full of healthy fats and carbs, they make an awesome entrée but also a fab snack. Give them a try!

Serves: 1
Time: 4 hours on low

Ingredients
- 1 poblano pepper
- 1/3 cup finely chopped cauliflower
- 1/3 lb. ground beef
- 1 tablespoon chopped onion
- 3 tablespoons tomato sauce
- 3 tablespoons shredded cheese
- Oil, to fry

Method
1. First, cut the poblano pepper in half and remove the seeds. Set to one side.
2. Warm some oil in a skillet and brown the ground beef. Remove from the heat and place into a large bowl.
3. Add the chopped cauliflower, tomato sauce and shredded cheese and stir well to combine.
4. Stuff the mixture into the pepper shell and place into your slow cooker.
5. Add a small amount of water to the bottom of your slow cooker, replace the lid and cook on low until 4 hours.
6. Serve and enjoy!

Homemade Keto Meatloaf with Goat's Cheese and Spinach

Feeling hungry? Then make sure you add this meatloaf to the menu. I've added it here to the appetizers section as it makes a perfect party nibble, or starter, but feel free to pile it onto your place and enjoy it as part of your main course.

Serves: 4-8
Time: 4 hours

Ingredients

- 2lbs (450g) fatty ground beef
- 2 free range eggs
- 3 scallions, chopped
- 1 large onion, chopped
- 3 cloves garlic, finely chopped
- handful of raw baby spinach
- 3-4 oz. (110g) goat's cheese
- 2 tablespoons tomato paste
- 4 shakes of cayenne pepper
- ½ teaspoon dried oregano
- 1 sprigs of rosemary
- Salt and pepper to taste

Method

1. First, grease your slow cooker with butter or oil. Set to one side.
2. Place the meat into a large bowl along with the eggs, the scallions, onion and the garlic. Mix well to combine.
3. Next add your spices- throw in the cayenne, oregano, salt and pepper and mix it all up again.
4. Place some plastic wrap onto the counter and place the meat on top. Flatten gently until it forms a long rectangle.
5. Place the spinach leaves and goat cheese right the in the middle then using one side of the plastic wrap, roll into a cylinder.
6. Spread with tomato paste (if using), sprinkle with rosemary and more salt and pepper.
7. Place into the slow cooker and cook on low for around 4 hours until cooked through.
8. Serve and enjoy!

Buffalo Chicken Cream Cheese Fondue

For those days when you want an appetizer with a difference and you really want to impress your friends and family, create this creamy, spicy fondue which is flecked with succulent chicken pieces and is almost completely hands-off.

Serves: 2-4
Time: 10-15 mins approx.

Ingredients
- 16oz (450g) cream cheese
- 1 cup (300ml) Frank's Red-Hot Sauce
- 1 cup (300ml) sugar-free ranch dressing
- 1 1/2 cups (150g) shredded cheddar
- 4 cups (500g) shredded chicken

Method
I love the simplicity of this one.
1. Simply throw all the ingredients into the slow cooker and warm on a low heat until everything has melted.
2. Give it all a good stir then serve!

Garlicky Shrimp

Shrimp gently flavored with garlic and red pepper. What's there not to like? Besides, these are extra-fast to prepare and make the most delicious hands-off starter in the world! Enjoy!

Serves: 6 - 8
Time: 40 mins- 1 hour

Ingredients

- 3/4 cup (180ml) olive oil
- 6 cloves garlic, thinly sliced
- 1 teaspoon smoked Spanish paprika
- 1 teaspoon kosher salt
- 1/4 teaspoon freshly ground black pepper
- 1/4 teaspoon crushed red pepper flakes
- 2 lbs. (900g) raw shrimp, peeled and deveined
- 1 tablespoon minced flat-leaf parsley, for garnish

Method

1. Open up the slow cooker and place inside the oil, garlic, paprika, salt, pepper and red pepper then give it a good stir to mix.
2. Cover and cook on high for about 30 minutes.
3. Remove the lid and place the shrimp inside.
4. Cover again and cook on high for 15-30 minutes. Check throughout to make sure they're cooking.
5. Serve on a plate with a generous serving of the sauce, then sprinkle with parsley and enjoy!

Sour Cream and Horseradish Cheese Dip

I love this one served with multiseed crackers or low carb veggies as a quick snack, appetizer or even as the centerpiece for a buffer at a party. You can make massive quantities of the stuff to keep you going when there's a game on. Awesome!

Serves: loads!
Time: less than 30 minutes

Ingredients
- 8 oz. (225g) cream cheese
- 8 oz. (225g) Pub Cheese
- 8 oz. (225g) sour cream
- 1 tablespoon red wine (optional)
- 1 teaspoon horseradish
- 1/4 teaspoon garlic powder
- 1/4 teaspoon onion powder
- Dash of onion salt to taste

Method
Another really easy one.
1. Simply place all the ingredients into your slow cooker
2. Turn the heat as low as possible and gently warm, stirring constantly until all the ingredients combine.
3. Serve and enjoy!

NOTE: You don't want to be melting it completely- just enough to be soft, warm and yummy!

Breakfast

Ham, Ricotta and Spinach Breakfast Casserole

You know those mornings when you just want to grab something delicious to eat but you don't have time to be slaving away in the kitchen? That's when this awesome breakfast casserole will be your lifesaver. Simply throw it all together the night before and you have the perfect healthy breakfast or brunch that will keep the pounds falling off whilst also keeping your taste-buds happy. Here's how:

Serves: 15
Time: 7-8 hours on low

Ingredients
- 12 large free-range eggs
- ¼ cup (60ml) heavy whipping cream
- 1 cup (250g) ricotta cheese
- ½ small onion
- ¼ teaspoon salt
- ¼ teaspoon mixed herbs
- 1/8 teaspoon dried garlic
- 9 oz. (250g) frozen spinach, water squeezed out
- 1 lb. (450g) diced ham

Method
1. First chop that onion and place to one side.
2. Next take a large bowl and break into that the four eggs, the heavy whipping cream, the ricotta cheese and stir well to combine.
3. Throw in the onion you chopped earlier and give it another nice stir then place to one side.
4. Grab another bowl and in this, whisk together the rest of the eggs. Then combine both egg mixtures and mix together well.
5. Stir in the seasoning then the spinach and finally the diced ham.
6. Grease your slow cooker with your favorite oil and pour the batter into the pan.
7. Replace the lid then cook on low for around 7-8 hours or overnight.

Slow Cooker Spinach & Feta Quiche

Let's be honest. There comes a point where you're a little tired of eating eggs, bacon and sausages for breakfast. Well, I have great news! This succulent and satisfying spinach and feta quiche provides you the same fat-burning benefits ingredients but with even more flavor!! Can you believe it?

Serves: 8
Time: 7-8 hours on low

Ingredients
- 8 eggs
- 2 cups (480ml) milk
- 2 cups (60g) fresh spinach
- 2 cloves garlic, minced
- 1/2 cup (50g) shredded Parmesan cheese
- 3/4 cup (100g) feta cheese, crumbled
- 1/4 cup (25g) shredded cheddar cheese
- Salt and Pepper to taste

Method
1. Take a large bowl and break into it the eggs then pour in the milk and whisk well to combine.
2. Next throw in the spinach, garlic, feta, parmesan and seasoning and stir well to mix.
3. Grease your slow cooker with your favorite oil then pour the batter in on top.
4. Sprinkle the cheddar cheese over the top, pop the lid back on and cook on low for 7-8 hours or overnight.

Keto Blueberry Breakfast Pancakes

There's nothing like the smell of blueberry pancakes in the morning to really wake up your stomach and give you that dose of energy you deserve. Try these light, fluffy ones. You'll never believe that they're Keto.

Serves: 4
Time: less than 30 minutes

Ingredients
- 3 large free-range eggs
- ¾ cup (190g) ricotta
- ½ teaspoon vanilla extract
- ¼ cup (60ml) milk
- 1 cup (100g) almond flour
- ½ cup (55g) golden flaxseed meal
- ¼ teaspoon salt
- 1 teaspoon baking powder
- ¼-½ teaspoon stevia powder
- ¼ cup (40g) blueberries

Method
1. First, take a large bowl and whisk together the eggs, ricotta, vanilla extract and milk. Set to one side.
2. In a separate bowl, mix the dry ingredients and stir well to combine. Then add the dry ingredients into the wet and stir well until a smooth batter forms.
3. Now, switch on your slow cooker and turn the heat up to high. Grease with the oil of your choice. When it's nice and hot, drop in the batter, add 3-4 blueberries per pancake (if using) and flip over to cook on both sides.
4. Remove, stack up and repeat until of the batter has been used.
5. Serve and enjoy!

Keto Breakfast Brownies

I love the fact that when you go Keto, you can keep enjoying foods that you'd think of as 'naughty' even when you're losing weight! It's awesome! And best of all, provided you stick to the diet guidelines, you keen on losing weight, even if you eat chocolate brownies for breakfast....

Serves: 6
Time: 1 hour approx.

Ingredients

- 1 cup (110g) golden flaxseed meal
- ¼ cup (25g) cocoa powder
- 1 tablespoon cinnamon
- ½ tablespoon baking powder
- ½ teaspoon salt
- 1 large egg
- 2 tablespoons coconut oil
- ¼ cup (80g) sugar-free caramel syrup
- ½ cup (112g) pumpkin puree
- 1 teaspoon vanilla extract
- 1 teaspoon apple cider vinegar
- ¼ cup (30g) slivered almonds

Method

1. Take a large mixing bowl and throw in all the dry ingredients. Give it a stir to combine.
2. In a separate bowl, throw together the wet ingredients and give them a nice stir to combine too.
3. Next pour the wet into the dry and mix well to combine. Resist the urge to over-stir here- a few clumps and lumps are fine!
4. Now you need to decide on how you're planning to cook your muffins. You can either use the special insert that your slow cooker manufacturer might have provided, find one in your own stash that will fit inside or simply make a large brownie-style cake directly in the bottom. Whatever you decide, make sure it's greased and ready to go
5. Pour the batter into the vessel and cook until the batter springs back to the touch- if you're using individual cakes, this should take between 15-30 minutes on high or 30 mins - 1 hour on low.
6. Serve and enjoy!

Spinach and Sausage Breakfast Frittata

I really love the simplicity of this recipe. It also provides all your major nutrients and is ready super-quick. Pop it on before you wake for your morning run and you'll have it ready for when you get home. (Tip: Try cooking it on high for 1-11/2 hours for an even faster version).

Serves: 4
Time: 2-3 hours approx.

Ingredients
- ¾ cups (120g) frozen spinach, defrosted
- 1 ½ cups (250g) diced red bell pepper (opt)
- ¼ cups (35g) diced red onion
- 8 free-range eggs
- Salt and pepper to taste
- 1 ⅓ cups (170g) cooked sausage

Method
1. Grab a bowl and combine the frozen spinach, the red pepper (if using), the red onion, the eggs, the seasoning and the sausage and stir well to combine
2. Grease your slow cooker with the oil of your choice and pour the batter inside.
3. Cook on low for 2-3 hours until set then serve and enjoy!

Jalapeño Popper Egg Cups

Ready for a perfectly portable breakfast with some real flavor that will please your taste-buds and light up your digestive system? Of course you are! Create these, jump into the shower and you'll have an awesome Keto breakfast waiting for you.

Serves: 2-4
Time: 30-45 mins

Ingredients
- 4 oz. (115g) cheddar cheese
- 3 oz. (85g) cream cheese
- 4 medium jalapeño peppers, de-seeded and chopped
- 12 strips bacon, cooked
- 8 large free-range eggs
- ½ teaspoon garlic powder
- ½ teaspoon onion powder
- Salt and pepper to taste

Method
1. Take a large bowl and mix together the eggs, cream cheese, the jalapeno, the garlic powder, the onion powder and the salt and pepper.
2. Now grease the inside of whatever baking tin you decide to use, whether that's the tin the manufacturer provided or just a regular tin that fits inside your slow cooker.
3. Pour the batter into the tin and place the bacon around the edges of each one followed by a nice handful of the cheese. Place into your slow cooker, replacing the lid carefully and cook on high for 30 mins approx.
4. Remove from the oven to cool and then enjoy!

Cinnamon Roll Oatmeal

Missing your morning dose of warm and comforting oatmeal? Then you'll LOVE this Keto version. Perfectly spiced with cinnamon and with the added crunch of crushed pecans you'll be set and ready for the day.

Serves: 6
Time: 30 mins - 1 hour

Ingredients
- 1 cup (125g) crushed pecans
- 1/3 cup (40g) flax seed meal
- 1/3 cup (55g) chia seeds
- 3 oz. (85g) cauliflower, finely chopped or blended into 'rice'
- 3 ½ cups (826ml) coconut milk
- ¼ cup (60ml) heavy cream
- 3 oz. (85g) cream cheese
- 3 tablespoons butter
- 1 ½ teaspoons cinnamon
- 1 teaspoon maple flavor
- ½ teaspoon vanilla extract
- ¼ teaspoon nutmeg
- ¼ teaspoon allspice
- 3 tablespoons erythritol, powdered
- 10-15 drops liquid Stevia

Method
1. Let's start by toasting your crushed pecans. Pop them into a pan over a low heat, then add the cinnamon, the maple flavor, the vanilla, nutmeg and allspice.
2. Meanwhile, heat the coconut milk in your slow cooker then once warm, add the cauliflower and bring to a boil. Cook for 30 minutes to an hour on high.
3. Then let's add the erythritol and the stevia to the pan, along with the flaxseed and chia seed and mix well. It will start getting really thick at this point.
4. In a small bowl, mix together the cream, butter and cream cheese and stir well to combine.
5. Remove the cauliflower 'oatmeal' from the pan, sprinkle over the toasted pecan and swirl through the cream mixture.
6. Serve and enjoy!

Maple Pecan Fat Bomb Bars

These ultra-nourishing fat bomb bars are perfect for those morning when you just want to grab something and run. Combining flaxseeds, almonds and coconut oil, you'll enjoy a good dose of healthy fats and know your body is thanking you for it from the inside! Enjoy!

Serves: 12
Time: Cooking time of 1-2 hours, plus cooling time of 1-2 hours.

Ingredients

For the Keto maple syrup...
- 2 ¼ teaspoons coconut oil
- 1 tablespoon unsalted butter
- ¼ teaspoon xanthan gum
- ¼ cup (50g) powdered erythritol
- ¾ cup (180ml) water
- ½ teaspoon vanilla extract
- 2 teaspoons maple extract
- ½ teaspoon cinnamon

For the fat bombs...
- 2 cups (200g) pecan halves
- 1 cup (100g) almond flour
- ½ cup (56g) golden flaxseed meal
- ½ cup (30g) unsweetened shredded coconut
- 8 tablespoons coconut oil
- ¼ teaspoon liquid Stevia

Method

1. First, we need to make the Keto maple syrup. Take a heat-proof bowl and add to it the coconut oil, the butter and the xanthan gum. Pop into the microwave for between 30 seconds to 1 minute, until melted.
2. In a separate bowl, combine the cinnamon and erythritol and stir well to combine. Then slowly add the water and stir well. Next add the vanilla extract and the maple extract then stir well. Finally, mix together the oils with this cinnamon mix and microwave for a further 30 seconds to 1 minute.
3. Leave to cool whilst we put the other ingredients together for the bars.

4. Firstly, switch your slow cooker on high, grease and pop in 2 cups of pecan halves then close the lid and leave for around 10-15 minutes until they start smelling wonderful!

5. Remove the pecans from the oven then pop them into a plastic bag and crush. I like to leave some chunky bits to add extra texture to the bars, but this is really up to you.

6. Now take a bowl and add the almond flour, flaxseed, coconut and the crushed pecans. To this add the coconut oil, the liquid Stevia and ¼ cup of the maple syrup that you've just made. Mix together well until it sticks together and forms a dough.

7. Re-grease your slow cooker and press the fat bomb dough into the bottom, pressing down lightly so it reaches in to the corners.

8. Cook on high for 30 minutes – 1 hour or 1-2 hours on low. Bear in mind that this may vary, depending on your slow cooker so please check throughout.

9. Remove the pan from your slow cooker and allow to cool for at least 1 hour before popping into the fridge for another hour *then* cutting.

10. Enjoy!

Herby Bacon, Mozzarella and Mushroom Frittata

Try this herby, cheesy mushroom frittata to take your breakfast to a whole new level of awesome. The mushrooms are a fantastic source of the antioxidant selenium and are also rich in vitamin D which makes them an incredible addition to your Keto breakfast. Enjoy!

Serves: 6
Time: 6-8 hours or overnight

Ingredients
- 7 slices bacon, fried
- 1 tablespoon olive oil
- 5-6 large mushroom caps
- 2 tablespoons fresh parsley
- ½ cup (12g) chopped fresh basil
- 4 oz. (115g) fresh mozzarella, cubed
- 2 oz. (57g) hard goat cheese, grated
- 8-9 large free-range eggs
- ¼ cup (60ml) heavy cream
- ¼ cup (25g) parmesan cheese, grated
- Salt and pepper to taste

Method
1. Let's get chopping first. Cut the bacon into smaller pieces (to taste), chop the basil and slice those mushrooms into pieces.
2. Pop a small amount of oil into the bottom of your slow cooker, turn onto high and add the mushrooms. Stir well and cook lightly.
3. Meanwhile, prepare your eggs by breaking them into a large bowl and adding the cream, the parmesan and the seasoning. Whisk well to combine.
4. Now add the egg mixture to the softened mushrooms in the bottom of the slow cooker, sprinkle over the mozzarella cheese, grate the goats cheese over the top of it all and replace the lid.
5. Cook for 30 minutes to 1 hour on high until set, or 1-1.30 hours on low. Remember that slow cookers can vary so please check throughout.
6. Serve and enjoy!

Almond Crusted Keto Breakfast Quiche

Who'd have thought about quiche for breakfast before you went Keto? Not me! But it's incredibly filling, provides those essential fats and keeps you effortlessly losing weight. Check it out!

Serves: 6-8 hungry people
Time: 1-2 hours

For the almond crust...
- 1 ½ cups (150g) almond flour
- ¼ cup olive oil (+1 tsp. if needed)
- 1 teaspoon dried oregano
- ¼ teaspoon salt

For the quiche filling...
- 6 large free-range eggs
- 1 ½ cups (180g) cheddar cheese, shredded
- 1 medium green bell pepper
- 6 slices bacon, fried
- 1 teaspoon garlic
- 1 teaspoon Mrs. Dash Table Blend (opt)
- Salt and pepper to taste

Method
1. Find a large bowl and add the almond flour, oregano and salt. Pour in the olive oil and mix well to combine. It should start sticking together now- form into a bowl. Feel free to add a drop more olive oil if needed.
2. Now grease the pan of your slow cooker and press the crust mixture into the bottom. Cook on high for around 30 minutes with a slight gap in the lid.
3. Let's make the filling now. Break the eggs in to the bowl and add the rest of the filling mixture before stirring well. Pour this over the crust in the slow cooker and replace the lid (completely this time) and cook on high until the eggs have set. This should take between 30 minutes -1 hour.
4. Remove the pan from the heat and allow to cool before slicing.
5. Serve and enjoy!

Chorizo-Cheese Breakfast Pie

Everyone loves pie for breakfast, don't they? Especially if it boasts the addition of spicy, succulent chorizo sausages! This one tastes great, keeps your weight-loss ticking away nicely and is super-easy to make. Just try!

Serves: 2
Time: 1-2 hours

Ingredients
- 2 chorizo sausages, sliced
- ¾ cup (95g) grated cheddar cheese
- ¼ cup (28g) coconut flour
- ¼ cup (50g) coconut oil
- 2 tablespoons water
- 5 large free-range egg yolks
- 2 teaspoons lemon juice
- ½ teaspoon rosemary
- ¼ teaspoon baking soda
- 1/8 teaspoon kosher salt

Method
1. Switch on your slow cooker, turn it up to high and add some oil. Gently fry the chorizo until browned, then set aside.
2. In a separate bowl, add the coconut flour, rosemary, cayenne pepper, baking powder and salt and place to one side.
3. Grab another bowl and beat those egg yolks until creamy. To this add the coconut oil, the water and the lemon juice and beat again.
4. Add the wet ingredients into the dry ingredients and mix again. Throw in the shredded cheese and stir through.
5. Now it's cooking time, but it's up to you how to do it. Either use the bowl of your slow cooker and pour the egg mixture over the top, or use the ramekin tin the manufacturer provided (or use your own, provided it fits!) Don't forget to add the chorizo.
6. Replace the lid and cook for 30 minutes on high or 1-2 hours on low.
7. Serve and enjoy!

Keto Breakfast Cheese and Bacon Tacos

Bet you didn't think it was possible to eat tacos and stick to a Keto diet, but you absolutely can. These amazing bacon tacos will fuel you right through your morning and keep you feeling great!

Servings: 3
Time: 30 minutes to 1 hour

Ingredients
- 1 cup (125g) shredded mozzarella cheese
- 6 large free-range eggs
- 2 tablespoons butter
- 3 strips bacon
- ½ small avocado
- 1 oz. (28g) shredded cheddar cheese
- Salt and pepper to taste

Method
1. Start by gently cooking the bacon in a skillet or inside your slow cooker until brown then set to one side.
2. Grease your slow cooker, turn the heat to high and sprinkle 1/3 (40g) cup mozzarella into the pan to form a circle shape. Once the corners start to brown, flip and cook on the other side. This is your first taco shell. Remove from the heat and hang over a wooden spoon resting on a pot.
3. Repeat with the rest of the mixture.
4. Now add the butter to the slow cooker then break the eggs into the cooker and cook on high. Stir well as they cook then gently spoon into the taco shells.
5. Top with sliced avocado, bacon, cheddar cheese and lashings of chili sauce.
6. Eat and enjoy!

Soups & Stews

Ground Beef Minestrone Soup

I'm the world's biggest fan of soup, and I don't just eat it when the temperatures drop but pretty much all year around. It's easy to make and it's just so yum! This beef minestrone soup certainly delivers! If you're strictly following Keto, feel free to omit the carrot. Enjoy!

Serves: 4
Time: 5-8 hours

Ingredients
- 1 lb. (450g) ground beef
- 2 small zucchinis, diced
- 1 yellow onion, diced
- 1 carrot diced
- 1 stalk of celery diced
- 1/2 cup (118ml) vegetable broth
- 3 cups (700ml) water
- 1 x 28 oz. (800g) can diced tomatoes
- 1 tablespoon minced garlic
- 1/2 teaspoon dried oregano
- 1/2 teaspoon dried basil
- Butter or oil for frying

Method
1. Take a large pan, add the oil or butter then add the ground beef. Cook gently until browned.
2. Next place into your slow cooker with the rest of the ingredients and cook on low for 5 to 8 hours.
3. Serve and enjoy

Thai Chicken Soup

Forget dull chicken soup that won't impress anyone and try this incredibly Asian-inspired soup instead. Infused with lemongrass, ginger and lime and beautifully simple, it will become one of your go-to recipes.

Serves: 4
Takes: 8-10 hours or overnight

Ingredients
- 1 whole chicken, chopped into chunks
- 1 stalk of lemongrass, cut into large chunks
- 20 fresh basil leaves (10 for the slow cooker, and 10 for garnish)
- 5 thick slices of fresh ginger
- 1 lime
- Salt and pepper to taste

Method
This one is super-easy.
1. Simply place the chicken, lemongrass, 10 basil leaves, ginger and seasoning into your slow cooker, cover with enough water to make soup* and cook on low for 8-10 hours or overnight.
2. When cooking time is over, pour into bowls, squeeze over lime and decorate with extra basil leaves.
3. Enjoy!

The exact amount you use is completely up to you. I like to just cover the vegetables but you might prefer to use more. Feel free to experiment!

Lentil and Italian Sausage Soup

If you love Italian sausages and you love soup, you'll adore this recipe! Featuring plenty of low carb veggies, this one is perfect for keeping you, erm... 'regular'. If you're strict with your carbs, you might want to skip the lentils or carrot, but rest assured, it will still be mind-blowingly yummy!

Serves: 6-8
Time: 6-8 hours or overnight

Ingredients
- 1 ½ lb. (680g) Italian sausage
- 2 teaspoons butter
- 2 teaspoons olive oil
- 5 cups (1.2 liters) chicken stock
- 1 1/2 (300g) cups lentils
- 1 cup (30g) spinach, packed
- 1/2 cup (75g) carrots, diced
- 1/2 cup (75g) onion, diced
- 4 cloves garlic, minced
- 1 small leek, cleaned and trimmed
- 1 rib celery, diced
- 1 cup (240ml) heavy cream
- 1/2 cup (60g) Parmesan cheese, grated
- 2 tablespoons Dijon mustard
- 2 tablespoons red wine vinegar
- Sea salt and black pepper, to taste

Method
1. Grab a large skillet, add the olive oil and butter and brown the sausage.
2. Remove the sausage and add to the bottom of your slow cooker along with the cooking fat.
3. Next rinse the lentils, if using and add to slow cooker, followed by the spinach, carrots, onions, garlic, leek, celery and seasoning, followed by the stock.
4. Finally add the cream, parmesan, Dijon mustard and red wine vinegar, stir well to mix and cook on low for 6-8 hours.
5. Serve and enjoy!

Creamy Reuben Soup

This amazing soup is just like the deli sandwich, but without any of those crazy carbs. Just taste it- you'll be impressed!

Serves: 6
Time: 4-6 hours on low or 6-8 hours on high.

Ingredients
- 1 medium onion, diced
- 2 ribs celery, diced
- 2 large cloves garlic, minced
- 3 tablespoons butter
- 1 lb. (450g) corned beef, chopped
- 4 cups (950ml) beef stock
- 1 cup (150g) sauerkraut
- 1 teaspoon caraway seeds
- 2 cups (480ml) heavy cream
- 1 ½ cup (185g) Swiss cheese, shredded
- Salt and pepper to taste

Method
1. Start by adding the butter to your slow cooker, turning the heat up to high and add the onion, celery, garlic and butter. Once these veggies are nice and soft, add the rest of the ingredients, except the cream and cheese and cook on high for 4-5 hours or low for 6-8 hours.
2. An hour before serving, stir through the heavy cream and cheese and cook for an extra hour on high.
3. Serve and enjoy!

Spicy Jambalaya Soup

Are you ready for a dose of Creole? Fancy spicy Keto goodness that will make your mouth water and fill you with a ton of nutrition? Your wish is my command.

Serves: 4-6
Time: 6-8 hours

Ingredients

- 5 cups (1.2 liters) chicken stock
- 2 tablespoons oil or butter
- 4 bell peppers, chopped
- 1 large onion, chopped
- 1 large can diced tomatoes with juice
- 2 cloves garlic, diced
- 2 bay leaves
- 1 lb. (453g) large shrimp, raw and de-veined.
- 4 oz. (115g) chicken, diced
- 1 package spicy Andouille sausage
- ½ head cauliflower
- 2 cups (200g) okra
- 3 tablespoons Cajun Seasoning (see recipe here)
- 4 tablespoons spicy sauce

Method

1. Firstly, heat the oil in your slow cooker and add the chopped peppers, onions, garlic and chicken. Stir well and allow to gently brown for 5 minutes.
2. Next add the Cajun seasoning, hot sauce and bay leaves, followed by the chicken stock. Replace the lid and cook on low for 6-8 hours or overnight.
3. Just before the end, chop the sausages into bite-sized pieces and add to the slow cooker.
4. Meanwhile, place the cauliflower into a food processor and pulse until it forms rice. Add to the slow cooker along with the raw shrimp.
5. Eat and enjoy!

Chicken and Kale Soup

Sometimes simple is best, especially when it comes to chicken soup. Give this chicken soup and try and you'll see what I mean! The added butter enriches the soup, ups the fats and also helps you absorb maximum minerals from that kale- awesome! Feel free to omit the carrots if you desire.

Serves: 4-6
Time: 6-8 hours or overnight

Ingredients
- 6 boneless, skinless chicken thighs or breasts
- 3 ½ cups (800ml) homemade chicken bone broth
- ½ large white onion, chopped
- 4 large cloves of garlic
- 1 ½ cups (75g) shredded carrots (opt)
- 4 cups (180g) chopped kale
- 1 ½ teaspoon parsley
- Salt and pepper to taste
- Butter, to taste

Method
1. Start by placing some butter in your slow cooker, turn the heat on and warm gently. Add the onions and the garlic and soften gently for five minutes.
2. Next add the chicken and the broth and cook for about 4-6 hours on low.
3. Then add the carrots, kale, parsley, salt and pepper and cook for an extra hour.
4. Serve and enjoy!

Cheesy Cauliflower Soup

This cheesy cauliflower soup is totally the bomb! It takes me through every single winter season and ensures I have all the fats I need to stick to my Keto plan, plus hit that comfort food zone nicely. I've said it will serve 6-8 but feel free to double up and enjoy more- this stuff is great for your body!

Serves: 6-8

Time: 4-6 hours

Ingredients

For the soup...
- 8 oz. (110g) butter
- 2 leeks, sliced and rinsed well
- 2 cloves garlic minced
- 8 oz. (110g) mushrooms
- 1 teaspoon Xanthan gum
- 4 cups (950ml) chicken broth
- 3 cups (975g) chopped cauliflower
- 2 cups (200g) shredded cheddar cheese plus extra for serving
- ½ cup (120ml) heavy cream
- Salt & pepper to taste

For the garnish...
- Shredded Cheddar Cheese
- Bacon crumbles
- Green onion
- Chili sauce

Method

1. Place the butter into your slow cooker, turn the heat up to high and add the cauliflower and leeks. Stir well and cook for about five minutes until they begin to soften.
2. Next add the mushrooms and cook for a further 2-3 minutes.
3. Add the chicken broth and stir well until everything is combined.
4. Replace the lid and cook on low for 4-6 hours.
5. At the end, remove the lid and stir in the cheese and the cream and allow it to sit until the cheese melts. Then stir in the xanthan gum until the soup thickens.
6. Season with salt and pepper then top with whatever toppings you desire.

Rosemary, Turkey and Kale Soup

Mmmmm! This easy soup is like eating a turkey roast dinner but in a bowl. Combining the rich flavor of turkey with fragrant rosemary and mineral rich, low carb spinach, you'll want to add this one to your go-to list. Enjoy!

Serves: 2-4
Time: 4-6 hours

Ingredients
- ½ tablespoon butter or lard
- ½ yellow onion, chopped
- 2-3 carrots, peeled and sliced
- 2 cloves garlic, pressed
- 3 cups (700ml) turkey stock
- 1-2 sprigs rosemary, each 2-4 inches in length
- 2 cups (250g) turkey meat, chopped into bite-sized pieces
- 2 cups (60g) spinach
- Salt and pepper, to taste

Method
1. Warm the fat in your slow cooker on a high heat and add the onion. Cook for five minutes until they soften.
2. Add the carrots and cook for 2-3 minutes, followed by the garlic, cooking for a further minute or two.
3. Season to taste then add the turkey stock, the turkey meat and the rosemary then cook over a low heat for 4-6 hours.
4. Stir through the spinach, remove the rosemary stems and then serve and enjoy!

Meat
Lemongrass and Coconut Chicken Drumsticks

I wanted to start this section with something a little different to really tease your taste buds and show you just how good Keto slow cooker food can be, and these Asian-inspired beauties certainly do the job. I waved my magic Keto wand on these by keeping the skin on the chicken and (serving with plenty of mayonnaise) but you might prefer to remove it beforehand- experiment and see what you love the best.

Serves: 2-3 approx.
Time: 4-5 hours

Ingredients
- 10 organic chicken drumsticks
- 1 thick stalk fresh lemongrass, papery outer skins and rough bottom removed, trimmed to the bottom 5 inches
- 4 cloves garlic, minced
- 1 thumb-size piece of ginger, thinly sliced
- 1 cup (235ml) coconut milk (+¼ cup optional at the end)
- 2 tablespoons fish sauce
- 3 tablespoons coconut aminos
- 1 teaspoon five spice powder
- 1 large onion, thinly sliced
- ¼ cup fresh scallions, chopped
- Salt and pepper to taste.

Method
1. Grab yourself a nice big bowl and place your drumsticks inside.
2. Remove the skins if that's what you're planning to do and season with salt and pepper to taste.
3. Place the ginger, garlic, lemongrass, fish sauce, coconut milk, coconut aminos and five spice powder into a high-speed blender and blitz until you form a smooth sauce.
4. Pour this into the bowl over the chicken and mix well.
5. Open up your slow cooker and layer the sliced onion over the bottom, followed by the drumsticks and marinade.
6. Turn onto low and cook for 4-5 hours. (don't overcook them!)
7. Serve and enjoy!

Best Jerk Chicken in the WORLD!

As you might already know if you've read my last book, I'm a massive fan of spicy food and so I adore these jerk chicken pieces. Super-easy and ready in a couple of hours, they make a perfect dinner or even a quick superbowl snack. Yum!

Serve: 2-4
Time: 5-6 hours

Ingredients
- 5 drumsticks and 5 wings
- 4 teaspoons salt
- 4 teaspoons paprika
- 1 teaspoon cayenne pepper
- 2 teaspoons onion powder
- 2 teaspoons thyme
- 2 teaspoons white pepper
- 2 teaspoons garlic powder
- 1 teaspoon black pepper

Method
1. Grab a large bowl and throw in all the spices and mix together well. If you're not a fan of spicy, leave out the cayenne and paprika, then add more onion powder instead.
2. Now place the chicken into the bowl and rub the spices into the chicken really well then place into the slow cooker.
3. Set the slow cooker on low and cook for 5-6 hours. You don't need any liquid here- the chicken contains enough already.
4. Cook until the chicken is perfect then serve and enjoy!

Mexican Crock Pot Fajita Chicken

Bring a taste of central America into your life by hopping in to the kitchen, throwing a bunch of ingredients into the slow cooker and returning a couple of hours late. How much easier do you want Keto cooking to be??

Serves: 4-6
Time: 6-8 hours

Ingredients

- 2lbs (907g) chicken breast, sliced thin
- 4 cloves garlic, minced
- 2 cups bell peppers, sliced
- 1 teaspoon kosher salt
- 1 teaspoon ground coriander
- 1 teaspoon dried oregano
- 1/2 teaspoon ground cumin
- 1/2 teaspoon chipotle chili powder
- 14oz (400g) can diced tomatoes

Method

This has to be the easiest recipe of all.

1. Just place your chicken into the bottom of your slow cooker, cover with the sliced onion, pepper and garlic and sprinkle the spices over the top.
2. Finally, pour over the diced tomatoes then cover with the lid and cook on low for 6-8 hours until cooked through.
3. Serve and enjoy!

Slow Cooker Roasted Chicken with Lemon Parsley Butter

Most of us adore roasted chicken, but we're not too keen on all of the cooking time and attention it needs when you do it in the oven. Not so when you use the power of your slow cooker. Simply prepare the bird, cook it for a couple of hours and return when it's nearly done. Easy!

Serves: 4-6
Time: 3 hours

Ingredients
- 1 whole chicken (5 – 6lbs/2.2kg-2.7kg)
- 1 cup (236ml) water
- 1/2 teaspoon salt
- 1/4 teaspoon ground black pepper
- 1 whole lemon, sliced thinly
- 4 tablespoons butter
- 2 tablespoons chopped fresh parsley

Method
1. Let's take care of the chicken first by removing any innards or stray feathers, then rub with salt and pepper.
2. Open up the slow cooker, place the chicken inside and pour the water over. If the water doesn't cover the bottom, add more.
3. Cook on high for around 3 hours until cooked through.
4. Then add the butter, parsley and lemon into the pot and return to the heat for 10 minutes.
5. Serve and enjoy!

Greek Chicken

When I was a child, we used to visit the beautiful Greek islands every year for our summer break and it was absolutely breath-taking! The food, the weather and the people completely stole my heart. That's why I love making this succulent and fragrant simple Greek chicken. Packed with flavor and easy to make, you'll be booking your trip before you know it!

Serves: 2-4
Times: 6-8 hours

Ingredients

- 3-4 boneless, skinless chicken breasts
- 2 tablespoons fresh garlic, minced
- Butter or lard, to grease
- 3 tablespoons lemon juice
- 1½ cups (350ml) hot water
- 2 chicken bouillon cubes
- 1 teaspoon dried oregano
- ½ teaspoon dried thyme
- ½ teaspoon dried mint
- ½ teaspoon dried basil
- ¼ teaspoon dried marjoram
- ½ teaspoon onion powder
- ¼ teaspoon garlic powder
- Salt and pepper to taste

Method

1. Start by greasing your slow cooker pan generously with butter or lard.
2. Place the spices into a large bowl and stir well to combine.
3. Take the chicken breasts, place onto a clean plate and rub each piece generously with the fresh garlic. I like to use about ½ tablespoon per piece.
4. Next place the chicken into the spice mixture and coat. Rub the spices into the flesh and ensure it all gets covered.
5. Open up the lid of your slow cooker and place the chicken breasts inside, followed by the lemon juice.
6. Dissolve the chicken bouillon cubes into the hot water and then pour over the chicken. Replace the lid and cook on low for 6-8 hours until cooked and tender.
7. Serve and enjoy!

Sesame- Orange Chicken

Orange chicken is a Chinese dish which usually comes deep fried, but we've given it a slow cooker makeover here. Thanks to the added butter, you still get those important fats but in a flavor-packed, easy version that take the minimum of effort but still stick to those Keto principles. It's fragrant, it's very special and you'll adore the orange taste.

Serves: 4
Time: 6-8 hours

For the chicken...
- ¼ cup melted coconut oil
- ¼ cup coconut milk
- 2 tablespoons butter or lard
- 2 tablespoons erythritol
- 1 teaspoon toasted sesame oil
- 1 teaspoon soy sauce
- ½ teaspoon fresh ginger, grated
- ½ teaspoon toasted sesame seeds
- ½ teaspoon orange extract
- ¼ teaspoon fish sauce
- 1½ lbs. chicken legs or thighs

For the garnish...
- 1 tablespoon black sesame seeds
- 4 green onions, sliced

Method
1. First take a small bowl, add all the ingredients except the chicken and stir well until combined.
2. Then place the butter into the bottom of your slow cooker, followed by the chicken pieces, then the sauce and replace the lid.
3. Cook on low for 6-8 hours or overnight until tender.
4. Serve and enjoy!

Italian Zucchini Meatloaf

The Italians really know their food, and boy, do they know how to do meatloaf! With fresh beef, juicy zucchini and utterly delicious herbs, everyone in your family will love this one. Try it now!

Serves: 6-8
Time: 3-4 hours

Ingredients
For the meatloaf...
- Olive oil or butter
- 2 lbs. (900g) ground sirloin
- 2 large free-range eggs
- 1 medium size zucchini, grated and excess liquid squeezed out
- 1/2 cup (60g) freshly grated Parmesan cheese
- 1/2 cup (12g) fresh parsley, chopped
- 4 cloves garlic, minced
- 3 tablespoons balsamic vinegar
- 1 tablespoon dried oregano
- 2 tablespoons onion powder
- 1/2 teaspoon sea salt
- 1/2 teaspoon ground black pepper

For the topping...
- 1/4 cup (55g) tomato sauce
- 1/4 cup (40g) shredded mozzarella cheese
- 2 tablespoons fresh parsley, chopped

Method
1. Place a large sheet of aluminum foil into the bottom of your slow cooker then grease well with the olive oil or butter.
2. Then grab a large bowl and throw in all the meatloaf ingredients then mix well to combine. Don't worry if it seems wet- it's supposed to be!
3. Place mixture into a slow cooker, forming an oblong shape. Replace the lid then cook on low for 6 hours.
4. Remove the lid then spread the tomato sauce over the top, followed by the cheese. Replace the lid and leave for 10 minutes until the cheese has melted.
5. Remove from the slow cooker using the foil, then slice, serve and enjoy!

Chinese 5-Spice Pork Ribs

Gotta love these spiced pork ribs! You can get all caveman (or woman) and tear them from the bone whilst mopping the incredibly delicious juice from your skin and coming back again and again for more. Best of all, they'll help you keep shifting that weight. Awesome!

Serves: 4-6 hungry people
Time: 6-8 hours

Ingredients
- 3 lbs. (1.36kg) baby back pork ribs
- Salt and pepper to taste
- 2 teaspoons Chinese five-spice powder
- 3/4 teaspoon coarse (granulated) garlic powder
- 1 fresh jalapeño, cut into rings
- 2 tablespoons rice vinegar
- 2 tablespoons coconut aminos (or soy sauce)
- 1 tablespoon tomato paste

Method
1. Start by cutting the ribs in the pieces so they'll fit into the slow cooker. Then sprinkle with salt and pepper and massage in.
2. Next take a small bowl and in it, combine the Chinese 5-spice mixture and garlic and massage into the meat.
3. Place the jalapeño rings into the bottom of your slow cooker, followed by the rice vinegar, the coconut aminos and the tomato paste and stir it all together until combined.
4. Next add the ribs but stand them up, pop the lid back on and cook for 6-8 hours on high.
5. Cook until the ribs almost fall apart.

Pork Stew with Oyster Mushrooms

Don't be thinking that this is just your regular pork stew- it's soo much better than any I've ever tried before! Creamy and coconutty, laced with tender mushrooms and injected with flavor, it will keep your tummy full whilst keeping the weight off.

Serves: 4
Time: 6-8 hours

Ingredients
- 2 tablespoons butter or lard
- 1 medium onion, chopped
- 1 clove garlic, chopped
- 2lbs (900g) pork loin, cut into 1" cubes and patted dry
- ½ teaspoon salt
- ½ teaspoon freshly cracked black pepper
- 2 tablespoons dried oregano
- 2 tablespoons dried mustard
- ½ teaspoon ground nutmeg
- 1½ cups (355ml) bone broth or stock
- 2 tablespoons white wine vinegar
- 2 lbs. (900g) oyster mushrooms
- ¼ cup (60ml) full-fat coconut milk
- ¼ cup (60ml) ghee
- 3 tablespoons capers

Method
1. Turn your slow cooker onto a high heat and melt the butter or lard. Next add the meat and cook well until brown on both sides. Don't forget that you don't have to do this all at once- batches works well too. Remove the meat but keep the juices in the bottom.
2. Next add some more fat and add the onions and garlic and cook for around 5 minutes until soft.
3. Add the oregano, mustard, nutmeg, broth and vinegar and stir well to combine. Then add the meat back into the pan then cover with the lid and cook for 6 hours on low.
4. Remove the lid, throw in the mushrooms and an extra cup of water and cook for a further 1-2 hours.
5. Whisk in the coconut milk, ghee and capers then serve and enjoy!

Chili Pulled Pork

If you want a crowd-pleaser that's easy to make and tastes simply out of this world, make sure you put this on the list. It's entirely Keto of course but you don't need to tell everyone that- simply serve and let them tuck in to the spiced, melt-in-the-mouth pork. Then just wait till they beg you for the recipe!!

Serves: 6-10
Time: 8-10 hours

Ingredients
- 4 1/2 lb. (2kg) pork butt / shoulder
- 2 tablespoons chili powder
- 1 tablespoon salt
- 1 ½ teaspoons ground cumin
- ½ teaspoon ground oregano
- ¼ teaspoon crushed red pepper flakes
- Pinch ground cloves
- ½ cup (120ml) stock or bone broth
- 1 bay leaf

Method
1. Start by grabbing a bowl and throwing in the chili, salt, cumin, oregano, red pepper flakes and pinch of cloves then stir well to combine.
2. Lay the pork out on a clean plate, remove the skin if applicable then rub the spice mixture into the pork. Place into the fridge and leave to marinade for 1-2 hours.
3. When you're ready to cook, pop the pork in the bottom of the slow cooker, add the bay leaf and the stock or broth, replace the lid and switch on. Cook on low for 8-10 hours (or overnight) until tender.
4. Remove the lid, lift the pork from the slow cooker and place onto a cutting board then shred with two forks.
5. Serve and enjoy!

Pork Chili Verde

Eating fabulous pork doesn't need to mean mixing spices, rubbing it all in and getting messy! This recipe takes just a handful of ingredients but still tastes amazing. I love to make this when I have friends coming over so I can focus on them instead of slaving away in the kitchen. Enjoy!

Serves: 4-6
Time: 6-8 hours or overnight

Ingredients
For the pork...
- 2 lbs. (900g) boneless, pork stewing meat, chopped
- 3 tablespoons butter
- 3 tablespoons cilantro, chopped finely
- 1½ cups (390g) salsa verde
- 5 cloves garlic, minced and divided.
- ¼ teaspoon sea salt

To serve...
- 1 tablespoons extra cilantro

Method
1. Place the butter into the bottom of your slow cooker and allow to melt on a high heat. Add the minced garlic and the cilantro and stir well.
2. Next add the cubed pork into the bottom of the pan of your slow cooker and stir well. Cook until just browned.
3. Pour the salsa verde into the crock pot and give it a good stir then cook on low for 6-8 hours.
4. Serve, sprinkle with extra cilantro and enjoy! Easy!

New Mexico Carne Adovada

Ready for some more spice? I was hoping you'd say that! Because I have another awesomely spiced pork recipe for you. It will tickle your taste buds and keep you coming back for more- I promise! Note- you'll need to make the sauce first in a pan but it's very much worth it!

Serves: 6-8
Time: 6-8 hours

Ingredients
- 3 lbs. (1.3kg) pork shoulder, cut into cubes
- 8 oz. (25g) dried New Mexican chilis, rinsed
- 2 cups (475ml) chicken or beef stock
- 1 onion, chopped
- 6 cloves garlic, chopped
- 2 teaspoons dried Mexican oregano
- 1 teaspoon ground cumin
- 1 teaspoon ground coriander
- 1 teaspoon salt
- 2 teaspoons apple cider vinegar

Method
1. Let's turn our attention to those chili peppers first. Open them up, remove the stems, remove the seeds and break them into small pieces. You can keep the seeds if you want some heavy spice, but I recommend you experiment with what you can take first!
2. Place the chilis into a saucepan with the rest of the ingredients except the pork and simmer over a low heat for around an hour until the flavors are well combined. Cook slightly then blend with an immersion blender. Add extra liquid if you like and strain if you want a completely smooth sauce (although I like to keep them all in).
3. Pour the sauce into a glass baking dish, cover with the sauce and pop into the fridge overnight, stirring occasionally.
4. Remove from the fridge and bring back to room temp before you start cooking.
5. Place into the bottom of your slow cooker and cook on low for 6-8 hours until lovely and tender.
6. Serve and enjoy!

Slow Cooker Beef Stroganoff

Beef stroganoff is something I always create when I'm feeling a little bit low on energy and low in spirits. There's something about the creamy fragranced sauce that hits the reset button and makes me feel awesome again. This version calls for regular cream but you can also substitute for coconut cream if you like- it certainly adds a different twist to the flavor.

Serves: 4-6 people
Time: 4-6 hours

Ingredients
- 2 lbs. (900g) beef stew meat
- Butter or lard
- 2 teaspoons salt
- 1/2 teaspoon black pepper
- 1 teaspoon garlic powder
- 2 teaspoons paprika
- 1 teaspoon thyme
- 1 teaspoon onion powder
- 8 oz. (225g) sliced mushrooms
- 1/2 onion, sliced
- 1/3 cup (80ml) heavy cream
- 2 teaspoons red wine vinegar

Method
1. Take a medium bowl and throw the spices into it. Stir well to combine, then add the meat pieces. Mix together well and make sure you're rubbing the spices into the meat.
2. Grease the bottom of your slow cooker with butter or lard (to taste) and place the sliced mushrooms and onion on top, followed by the beef. Replace the lid and cook for 4-5 hours on low.
3. Open the lid and add the cream, vinegar and salt and pepper, stir well, then replace the lid and cook for a further hour or so until perfect.
4. Serve and enjoy!

Beef, Bacon & Cabbage Stew

This rich stew provides all the healthy fat you need to keep that weight falling off whilst never compromising on taste. Flecked with nutrient-rich green cabbage and lifted with the addition of red onions and thyme, this makes the perfect winter meal for when you want easy and tasty.

Serves: 6-8
Time: 7-8 hours

Ingredients
- ½ lb. (225g) uncured bacon, cut into strips
- 3 lbs. (1.3kg) beef, cut into medium- pieces
- 2 large red onions, sliced
- 1 tablespoon butter
- 1 clove garlic, minced
- 1 small green or Savoy cabbage
- Salt and pepper to taste
- 1 sprig fresh thyme
- 1 cup beef bone broth or water

Method
1. Open your slow cooker (but don't turn on yet) and add the butter, followed by the bacon, the onion slices and the garlic
2. Next add the beef and surround with the cabbage slices.
3. Sprinkle everything with the thyme, pour over the broth, season with salt and pepper and pop that lid back on.
4. Cook on low for 7-8 hours until the meat is beautifully tender.

Sweet Pepper Beef Tongue

Beef tongue is something that isn't eaten so much these days but is definitely something you'll want to try. Packed with iron, zinc, vitamin B-12 and high levels of fat, it provides the perfect balance between health and taste. If you're strict about Keto, feel free to omit the peppers, but I recommend keeping them in for added flavor!

Serves: 6-8
Time: 3-6 hours

Ingredients
- 3lb (1.3kg) beef tongue
- 1 onion, quartered
- 1 onion, diced
- 1 green bell pepper, diced
- 1 yellow pepper, diced
- 2 Jalapeno Pepper, diced
- 6 cloves garlic, minced
- 2 teaspoons salt, divided
- 1 teaspoon pepper
- 1 teaspoon Cajun spice
- 8 oz. (225g) can tomato sauce
- 2 cups chicken stock or water)
- 1 ¾ sticks (200g) butter
- 1 bunch green onions

Method
1. First, we'll be cooking the tongue to perfect. Simply place into a large stock pot, cover with water, add a quartered onion, 1 teaspoon salt and simmer for about 3 hours until cooked.
2. Remove from the pan and cool until you can handle it. Peel off the skin then cut into cubes. Pop to one side.
3. Next open up your slow cooker and add approximately half of the butter. Melt over a high heat.
4. Add the onion, peppers, garlic and cook for about five minutes until they begin to soften. Add the remaining spices and cook for a further 1-2 minutes.
5. Add the chicken stock and the tomato sauce, followed by the chunks of tongue, replace the lid, turn down to low and cook for around 6 hours.
6. Once you're ready to serve, open the lid and melt over the rest of the butter.
7. Serve and enjoy!

Easy Slow Cooker Beef Chili

When the weather gets really bad outside, I love to curl up in the most comfortable chair in the house with a bowl of this amazing chili (topped with extra chili sauce, of course!) It will keep your digestion healthy, your taste buds happy and will ensure you can fit into your best party clothes this Thanksgiving.

Serves: 4-6
Time: 6-8 hours

Ingredients

- 2 ½ lbs. (1.1kg) ground beef
- 1 medium red onion, chopped and divided
- 4 tablespoons garlic, minced
- 3 large ribs of celery, diced
- 2 tablespoons butter, lard or oil
- ¼ cup (25g) pickled jalapeno slices
- 6 oz. (170g) can tomato paste
- 14oz (400g) can tomatoes and green chilies
- 14oz (400g) can stewed tomatoes with Mexican seasoning
- 2 tablespoons Worcestershire sauce
- 4 tablespoons chili powder
- 2 tablespoons cumin
- 2 teaspoons sea salt
- 1/2 teaspoon cayenne
- 1 teaspoon garlic powder
- 1 teaspoon onion powder
- 1 teaspoon oregano
- 1 teaspoon black pepper
- 1 bay leaf

Method

1. Firstly, add the butter, oil or lard to your slow cooker and turn onto a high heat. Add half the onions and cook for 5 minutes until softens. Add the garlic and cook for a further minute.
2. Add the beef to the onion mixture and cook until browned, stirring often. Heat slow cooker on low setting.
3. Then throw in the rest of the ingredients, give it all a stir to make sure it's well combined and replace the lid.
4. Cook on low for 6-8 hours or overnight.
5. Serve and enjoy!

Coconut & Broccoli Chicken Curry

There's something incredible about the way that coconut and chicken work together in curry- you get all the flavor and spicy goodness with a creamy and exotic edge. It's soo satisfying. Mmmmm...I'm going to have to make it now!

Serves: 2-4
Time: 6 hours

Ingredients

- 13 oz. (370ml) can coconut milk
- 1 lb. (450g) chicken thighs, chopped into bite-sized chunks
- 2 tablespoons curry paste
- 12 oz. (340g) broccoli florets
- 1 medium carrot, shredded (optional)
- 1 bell pepper, sliced in strips
- 1 handful fresh cilantro, chopped
- Salt and pepper, to taste

Method

1. This chicken curry is soo easy! Start by pouring the coconut milk into your slow cooker, followed by the curry paste. Stir to combine well, then add the chopped chicken, pop on the lid and cook on low for 4 hours.
2. Open up that lid and add the broccoli, carrots (if using) and pepper and cook for another hour with the lid on.
3. Remove the lid and check the consistency. If it seems a bit too thin, turn the heat up to high and cook for a further hour with the lid of.
4. Season with salt and pepper, top with cilantro and enjoy!

Easy Keto Ranch Chicken

This Keto ranch chicken is so incredibly easy and ready so incredibly fast that I promise you'll be creating it time and time again. Creamy and succulent, it only takes four ingredients and you'll have an unforgettable dish on your hands.

Serves: 6
Time: 4 hours

Ingredients
- 2 lbs. (900g) chicken breasts
- 3 tablespoons butter
- 4 oz. (115g) cream cheese
- 3 tablespoons dry ranch dressing mix

Method
1. Take the lid off your slow cooker and place the chicken right there inside with 2 tablespoons water.
2. Cut the cream cheese and the butter into chunks and smear over the chicken, followed by the range dressing mix.
3. Pop the lid on top then cook on high for 3-4 hours (or low for 5-7 hours)
4. Remove the lid, shred the chicken and enjoy!

Spiced Oxtail Stew

When was the last time you ate oxtail? I'm guessing that it was almost never. But oxtail is actually a perfect source of electrolytes, healthy fats and collagen which help keep you looking young and vibrant. And did I mention that it's really yummy too?

Serves: 4
Time: 4-6 hours

Ingredients

- 4.4lb (2 kg) oxtail or beef suitable for slow cooking (bones included)
- 1 tablespoon ghee, butter or lard
- 2 cups (480ml) beef stock
- 1 red onion, peeled and halved
- 1 garlic head
- 1 carrot
- 2 celery stalks
- Juice and peel from an orange
- 1 cinnamon stick
- 1/4 teaspoon nutmeg
- 5-8 cloves
- 1 x star anise
- 2 bay leaves
- Salt and pepper
- 4 heads small lettuce

Method

1. Start by opening up your slow cooker and placing the butter, ghee or lard inside. Switch on the heat, add the oxtail and brown over a high heat.
2. Now add the red onion, the spices, the stock, the orange juice, the carrot and garlic heads, replace the heat and cook on high for a few minutes, then turn down the heat and cook for 4-6 hours until the meat is beautifully soft.
3. Remove from oven and allow to cool. (Get rid of the spices, the orange and veg or eat if you can't resist!)
4. Serve and enjoy!

Chicken Pad Thai with Zucchini Noodles

Don't worry- you can still eat Pad Thai even though you're following a Keto diet! And you know what? It tastes even better than the regular kind. Beautifully flavored and served with tender, nutrient-dense zucchini noodles, you'll LOVE these. Enjoy!

Serves: 4-6
Time: 4-6 hours

Ingredients
For the Pad Thai...
- 2 lb. (900g) chicken thighs or breasts
- 2 tablespoons butter or lard
- 2 medium zucchinis
- 1 large carrot
- 1 handful of bean sprouts (optional)
- 1 small bunch green onions
- 1 cup (240ml) coconut milk
- 1 cup (240ml) chicken stock
- 2 heaping tablespoons peanut butter
- 1 tablespoon soy sauce
- 2 teaspoon Fish Sauce
- 2 teaspoon ground ginger
- 2 cloves garlic, minced
- 1 teaspoon cayenne pepper
- 1 teaspoon red pepper flakes.
- Salt & Pepper, to taste

To garnish...
- Chopped cashews
- Chopped cilantro

Method

1. Warm the butter or lard in the bottom of your slow cooker, add the chicken and cook over a high heat until brown. This will give you a ton of flavor!
2. Now add the coconut milk and the stock and stir well to combine. Now add the peanut butter, the soy sauce, fish sauce, ginger, garlic, onions, cayenne and red pepper and stir well until combined.
3. Now turn the zucchinis into noodles using a spiralizer or vegetable peeler, shred the carrots, wash the bean sprouts and place into a bowl. Toss to mix.
4. Pile the veggie mix on top of the meat but try to avoid them touching the liquid- you want them steamed but not soggy!
5. Replace the lid and cook for 3-4 hours on low.
6. Open up that lid and first remove the veggies, followed by the chicken.
7. Cut the meat into smaller pieces then place over the noodles, followed by a scattering of green onions, cashews and chopped cilantro to make it look pretty and taste even more awesome.
8. Serve and enjoy!

Italian Hot Stuffed Peppers

You're probably thinking *"Eeeek! Peppers aren't Keto friendly!!"* but you'd be wrong. Because not only are they one of the most nutritious veggies out there (packed with antioxidants and vitamins), they're also surprisingly low in carbs and, in my humble opinion, taste extremely yummy!

Serves: 5
Time: 6 hours

Ingredients
- 1 lb. (450g) ground Italian hot sausage.
- 5 assorted bell peppers
- 2 tablespoons butter or lard
- 1/2 head of cauliflower, chopped into a 'rice' consistency
- 8 oz. (225g) can tomato paste
- 1 small white onion, diced
- 1/2 head garlic, minced
- 1 small handful fresh basil, minced
- 2 teaspoon dried oregano
- 2 teaspoon dried thyme

Method

1. Firstly, slice a tiny bit off the bottom of the peppers so they stand up by themselves. Then carefully cut the tops off (but keep them) and scoop out the seeds then place to one side.
2. Place the cauliflower rice into a large mixing bowl and add the garlic, basil, dried herbs and onions and mix well to combine.
3. Now place the butter or lard into the bottom of your slow cooker, turn up the heat and place your sausages inside. Cook gently until lightly browned to make it all extra-tasty.
4. Throw your browned sausage into the cauliflower, followed by the tomato paste and mix well.
5. Grab your peppers and gently scoop as much of the 'rice' mixture into the peppers as you can. Place them into your slow cooker, pop their lids on, replace the lid and cook for 6 hours on low or overnight. If you have some of the mixture left over, don't worry- you can always heat it up for a separate meal.
6. Serve and enjoy!

Easy Korean Short Ribs

Craving Asian? Then make these amazing Korean short ribs! The sauce is thick and satisfying, the ribs will melt in your mouth and you'll be in heaven. Enjoy!

Serves: 8
Time 6-8 hours

Ingredients
- ½ cup (120ml) soy sauce
- ⅓ cup (80ml) erythritol
- ¼ cup (60ml) sugar-free rice vinegar
- 2 cloves garlic, peeled and smashed
- 1 tablespoon grated fresh ginger
- ½ teaspoon crushed red pepper
- 4 lbs. (1.8kg) beef short ribs
- 1 green cabbage, quartered
- ½ teaspoon guar gum (thickener)
- 1 tablespoon sesame oil
- 4 scallions, thinly sliced

Method
1. Easy peasy! Place the soy sauce, erythritol, vinegar, garlic, ginger and red pepper into your slow cooker. Top with the short ribs followed by the cabbage then replace the lid.
2. Cook on low for 7-8 hours until the meat is tender.
3. Next place the cabbage and ribs onto a plate and turn your slow cooker up to high.
4. Grab a small bowl, add 1 tablespoon of water and add the guar gum. Whisk well until thickened. Then throw it all into the cooking liquid along with the sesame oil and cook until thick.
5. Spoon the sauce over the ribs, top with the scallions and serve!
6. Enjoy!

Deep Dish Cheese & Pepperoni Pizza with Cauliflower Crust

Oh yes! This recipe is about to make your day! Pizza was the food I craved the most when I first started the Keto diet so I was soo pleased to discover this brilliant recipe. Low carb, extra-yummy and perfect for weight-loss indulgence. Yum!

Serves: 1
Time: 3-4 hours

Ingredients
For the crust...
- 1 large head cauliflower
- 2 eggs, beaten
- ½ cup (60g) shredded Italian cheese
- 1 teaspoon dried Italian seasoning
- ¼ teaspoon salt
- 1 tablespoon butter or lard
- *For the topping...*
- ½ cup (110g) jarred Alfredo sauce
- Pepperoni sausage, to taste
- ½ bell pepper, chopped (opt.)
- 1½ cups (180g) Italian shredded cheese
- ½ teaspoon dried rosemary

Method
1. First, we need to prepare the cauliflower by roughly shopping to florets then into finer pieces so it resembles rice. You can also do this directly in your food processor.
2. Place into a bowl and add the eggs, cheese, seasoning and salt and mix well.
3. Grease your slow cooker with the butter or lard and place the cauliflower mixture into the pan. Press down with your fingers.
4. Next open up the tomato sauce and spread onto the top of your cauliflower base, then add the rosemary, the chopped pepperoni, the bell pepper if using and top with cheese.
5. Pop the lid back on but use a wooden spoon to prop it open slightly.
6. Cook on high for 2-4 hours until crust is cooked.
7. Turn off and leave to rest for 30 minutes.
8. Serve and enjoy!

Seafood
Slow Cooker Trout with Orange and Pecans

For a quick, healthy meal that is ready in less than an hour and tastes amazing, make this slow cooker trout. It's light, flakey and has a gentle citrus kick that adds that extra oomph. Enjoy!

Serves: 1
Time: 30 minutes -1 hour

Ingredients
- 1 large trout fillet
- 1 tablespoon olive oil
- Salt and pepper, to taste
- 1 tablespoon butter
- 1 orange, zested and juiced
- ½ cup pecans, chopped
- Parsley, to garnish

Method
1. Place the butter in the bottom of your slow cooker and turn up to high.
2. Take your trout and season with salt and pepper, then place into the slow cooker. Cook on both sides for just a minute or two.
3. Now pour the orange juice over the top of the fish and sprinkle over the pecan.
4. Cover and cook on high for just 30 minutes until the fish flakes beautifully.
5. Serve garnished with the parsley.

Moqueca – Brazilian Fish Stew

Moqueca is one of my favorite ways to enjoy fish! With a delicious Brazilian flavor, plenty of healthy fats and beautifully soft fish, you'll want to share this one with your friends. Actually...perhaps not

Serves: 4-6
Time: 3-4 hours

Ingredients
- 2 lbs. (900g) white fish fillets (halibut, swordfish, or cod), pin bones removed, cut into large portions
- 3 cloves garlic, minced
- 4 tablespoons lime or lemon juice
- Salt and pepper to taste
- Olive oil
- 1 cup (100g) chopped spring onion
- 1 bell pepper, chopped
- 2 cups (400g) chopped tomatoes
- 1 tablespoon sweet paprika
- Pinch red pepper flakes
- 1 large bunch of cilantro, chopped
- 14oz (400ml) can coconut milk

Method
1. Start by placing the fish onto a large clean plate and coat with the garlic and the lime juice. Sprinkle with salt and pepper and place into the fridge to rest.
2. Place the olive oil into the slow cooker, turn onto high and add the onion and peppers. Cook for 5 minutes, stirring well. Then add the garlic and cook for an extra minute.
3. Add the tomatoes and the green onions, the paprika, the pepper flakes and sprinkle with more salt. Stir in the cilantro, pop the lid on and leave for 5-10 minutes.
4. Now open up the slow cooker, place the fish on top, pour the coconut milk over the top and gently spoon some of the veggies over the fish.
5. Replace the lid, turn the heat to low and simmer for 3-4 hours.
6. Taste and see if you need to add more flavors. Squeeze in the lemon or lime juice then serve and enjoy.

Perfectly Poached Salmon

This poached salmon is moist, luscious and perfect for just about any meal. Containing tons of healthy omega fatty acids, useful amounts of the amino acid taurine, phosphorus and vitamin B6, it's like a vitamin & mineral pill on a plate. Enjoy!

Serves 4 to 6
Time: 1 – 1 ½ hours

Ingredients
For the salmon...
- 2 cups (480ml) water
- 1 cup (240ml) dry white wine
- 1 lemon, thinly sliced
- 1 shallot, thinly sliced
- 1 bay leaf
- 5-6 sprigs tarragon, dill, and/or Italian parsley
- 1 teaspoon black peppercorns
- 1 teaspoon salt
- 2 lbs. (900g) skin-on salmon
- Salt and pepper to taste

To serve...
- Lemon wedges
- Coarse sea salt
- Olive oil for serving

☐Method
1. Start by placing the water, wine, lemon, shallots, bay leaf, fresh herbs, peppercorns and salt into your slow cooker and cook on high for 30 minutes.
2. Place the salmon onto a clean place, season with salt and pepper on the skin side and place in the slow cooker (skin side down).
3. Replace the lid then cook on high for 45 minutes-1 hour, checking frequently.
4. Remove from the slow cooker and place onto a plate, pouring over extra olive oil and salt.
5. Serve and enjoy!

Shrimp Fra Diavolo

This classic Italian-American dish is inexpensive, mouth-wateringly good and will help fill you up with comforting flavors and Italian-style love. It's ready quickly and will help you feel energized and amazing!

Serves: 2-4
Time: 2-3 hours

Ingredients

- 2 tablespoons avocado oil (can substitute with olive oil)
- 1 medium onion, diced
- 3-5 cloves garlic, minced
- 1 teaspoon red pepper flakes
- 14 oz. (400g) chopped tomatoes
- 1 tablespoons Italian parsley, chopped
- ½ teaspoon freshly-ground black pepper
- 1lb (450g) medium shrimp, shelled

Method

1. Start by placing the oil into the slow cooker, turn the heat to high and add the onions. Cook for five minutes, stirring often.
2. Then add the garlic and red pepper and cook for an extra 1-2 minutes.
3. Next throw in the tomatoes, parsley and black pepper and cook on low for 2-3 hours.
4. Open up the slow cooker and throw in the shrimp, then cover again and cook for 15 minutes or so until the shrimp is cooked. Check often to see how it's doing.
5. Serve and enjoy!

Keto Fish & Cheddar Pie

My grandmother always used to make fish pie every Friday and proudly serve it alongside huge hunks of bread. Whilst bread is off the menu these days, I always honor her memory by whipping up this Keto-friendly fish pie and wowing the whole family. It's just as tasty as it sounds- give it a try.

Serves: 4-6
Time: 3-4 hours

Ingredients
- 4 large eggs, hard boiled
- 1 large cauliflower
- ¼ cup (55g) + 2 tablespoon butter
- 2-3 fillets white fish such as haddock or cod, skinless
- 2 fillets salmon (skin removed)
- 2 fillets mackerel (skin removed)
- 1 medium red onion
- 2 bay leaves
- ¼ teaspoon ground cloves
- 1 cup (240ml) heavy whipping cream
- ½ cup (120ml) water
- 1 teaspoon Dijon mustard
- ⅛ teaspoon ground nutmeg
- 1 cup + ½ cup (170g) cheddar cheese, shredded
- 4 tablespoon freshly chopped chives
- Fresh parsley, for garnish
- Salt and pepper, to taste

Method
1. Make sure your eggs are hard-boiled, if not, do that now!
2. Next let's prepare the cauliflower. First chop into florets, steam or boil until tender and pop into your blender. Pulse into smooth then set aside.
3. Meanwhile, let's poach that fish. Pour the water and cream into the slow cooker and add the fish, the onion, the bay leaves and the cloves.
4. Replace the lid, turn onto high and cook for 10-15 minutes until tender.

5. Take the fish out of the slow cooker and place onto a clean plate, and set aside. Now let's finish off that sauce.

6. Add the remaining butter and nutmeg and simmer for a few minutes until it starts to thicken. Stir through 1 cup of the shredded cheese.

7. Next pop the fish back into the slow cooker, followed by the halved eggs, and spoon some of the cream and cheese sauce over everything else.

8. Sprinkle with the fresh herbs then top with cauliflower mash. Finally place the rest of the cheese on top then replace the lid of the slow cooker.

9. Cook on high for 1-2 hours.

10. Serve and enjoy!

Note: You can also remove the slow cooker pan and place under a pre-heated grill to brown the cheese if you like.

Dessert

Mocha Pudding Cake

When you want to lose weight, one of the things you'll probably start missing most is rich gooey chocolate cakes and pudding. Not so with this amazing Mocha pudding cake! It's 100% Keto, filled with tons of nutrition and you will still lose weight! Yippee!

Serves: 4-6
Time: 3-4 hours

Ingredients
- ¾ cup (170g) + 1 tablespoon butter, cut into large chunks
- 2 oz. (45g) unsweetened chocolate, chopped
- ½ cup (120ml) heavy cream
- 2 tablespoons instant coffee
- 1 teaspoon vanilla extract
- 4 tablespoons unsweetened cocoa powder
- 1/3 cup (30g) almond flour
- 1/8 teaspoon salt
- 5 large free-range eggs
- 2/3 cup (65g) stevia or erythritol

Method
1. Start by opening up your slow cooker and placing all the butter inside, along with the unsweetened chocolate. Turn to high and stir well as it melts together, then turn off the heat.
2. Take a small bowl and add the heavy cream, coffee and vanilla and stir well to combine. Set aside.
3. Take another bowl and combine the almond flour, cocoa and salt. Set aside.
4. Grab your eggs, find yet another bowl and whisk well until thickens, then add your sweetener. Keep beating until the mixture turns pale yellow and nice and thick.
5. Slowly pour in the melted butter and chocolate mixture we made earlier and keep beating. Follow with the cocoa, almond flour and salt and keep mixing.
6. Next, add the cream, coffee and vanilla mixture and stir well until everything is combined.
7. Pour into the slow cooker, cover with a tea towel and place the lid on top of this. (The tea towel will absorb condensation and keep your cake yummy.
8. Cook on low for 2-4 hours until the center is still soft but the edges are more solid like cake. (Like when you make chocolate brownies).

95

Vanilla-Almond Keto Cheesecake

Everyone loves cheesecake, don't they? And this version takes even better than the original!! Crunchy almonds make a mouth-watering base, and the effortlessly good filling is AMAZING. Top with berries if you aren't strictly following Keto or simply enjoy as it is.

Serves: 4-6
Time: 2 -3 hours

Ingredients
For the crust...
- 1 cup of toasted almonds (unsalted) or pecans ground to a meal in a blender or food processor
- 2 tablespoons butter
- 1 free-range egg

For the filling...
- 1lb (450g) cream cheese
- 2 free-range eggs
- 1 teaspoon stevia
- 1 teaspoon vanilla extract
- 4 tablespoons heavy cream
- 1 tablespoon coconut flour

Method
1. Let's make the base first. Place the base ingredients into a bowl, stir well and then press into the bottom of a cheesecake tin.
2. In a separate bowl or in your blender, mix together the ingredients for the filling. Taste to make sure it's sweet enough and add extra stevia if required.
3. Pour the filling over the base and set to one side.
4. Open the lid of your slow cooker and pour in one cup of water, then carefully lower the cheesecake inside. Don't get water inside the cheesecake itself!
5. Turn to high and cook for 2-3 hours. Remove from the heat when the middle is set.
6. Serve and enjoy!

Almond & Raspberry Cream Cake

I know I say it time and time again, but it's so hard to believe that this light, sweet and utterly delicious cake is Keto. If you're strict about Keto, you can omit the raspberries, but I'd really encourage you to keep them in- they're very low carb and taste incredible.

Serves: 12
Time: 3-4 hours

Ingredients
For the cake...
- 1 ¼ cup (120g) almond flour
- ½ cup (100g) erythritol or stevia
- ½ cup (65g) coconut flour
- ¼ cup (25g) vanilla flavor protein powder
- 1 ½ teaspoon baking powder
- ¼ teaspoon salt
- 3 large free-range eggs
- 6 tablespoons butter, melted
- 2/3 cup (160ml) water
- ½ teaspoon vanilla extract

For the filling...
- 8 oz. (225g) cream cheese
- 1/3 cup (70g) erythritol or stevia
- 1 large free-range egg
- 2 tablespoons whipping cream
- 1 ½ cup (180g) fresh raspberries

Method
1. Start by greasing your slow cooker then set to one side.
2. Take a large bowl and add the almond flour, sweetener, coconut flour, protein powder, baking powder and salt. Mix well.
3. Make a well in the bottom and add the eggs, melted butter and water. Stir well until combined. Set aside.

4. Now let's make the filling. Place the cream cheese into a bowl with the sweetener and beat until combined well. Then add the egg, the whipping cream and the vanilla extract and stir again until combined.
5. Let's get it all into your slow cooker now. Place about ½ to 2/3 of the batter into the pan, then top with the cream cheese mixture, and sprinkle the raspberries over the top.
6. Bake on low for 3-4 hours until the middle has set and the edges are just golden.
7. Cool completely before serving.
8. Enjoy!

Fudgy Two-Layer Brownies

Everyone I know absolutely adores chocolate brownies, and I expect you do too. If so, let me tell you that you're going to think you've died and gone to heaven with these. Just make them and you'll see

Serves: 16
Time: 1-2 hours

Ingredients
For the brownie layer...
- 3.5oz (100g) extra dark chocolate (85% cocoa or more)
- 4 ½ oz. (125g) butter or coconut oil
- 3 large free-range eggs
- ½ teaspoon liquid stevia
- 1 cup (100g) almond flour
- ½ cup plus 1 tablespoon cocoa powder
- 2 tablespoons chia seeds, ground
- ½ teaspoon baking powder
- 1 teaspoon cream of tartar

For the chocolate layer...
- 1.8oz (50g) extra dark chocolate (85% cocoa or more)
- 2 tablespoons butter or coconut oil
- ¼ cup (60ml) heavy whipping cream

Method
1. First grease the pan of your slow cooker with a small amount of butter and place to one side. You can also place parchment paper at the bottom to help you get the brownies out at the end, although it's not essential.
2. Let's start by making the brownie mixture. Break the chocolate into small pieces, place with the butter in a small bowl and warm gently in the microwave until melted. Stir well together.
3. Grab a separate bowl and place into it the eggs and stevia and stir well to combine. Then beat in the chocolate until lovely and thick using a hand blender.
4. Next add each of the dry ingredients in turn, stirring with a spoon. Don't worry if the ingredients aren't perfectly mixed- it all adds to the texture of the brownies.

5. Pour the mixture into the slow cooker pan, pop a tea towel over the top to absorb the moisture and pop the lid on top of that.
6. Cook on low for 1-2 hours until firm in the middle but not entirely cooked. Remember- brownies will further harden when they're out of the 'oven' so err on the side of caution. Remove and allow to cook.
7. Then we can make the chocolate layer. Break the chocolate into a small bowl with the butter and gently warm the cream in a saucepan. Pour the cream over the chocolate and stir well until combined. It should start looking glossy and yum at this point.
8. Pour the chocolate layer over the brownies and leave to cool.
9. Serve and enjoy!

Lemon & Poppy Seed Cake

This incredibly moreish lemon cake is best served warm from your slow cooker with a large helping of cream, and preferably a warm sunny spot to sit, enjoy the indulgence and let it all slip down into your stomach. Share it if you dare!

Serves: 8
Time: 3-4 hours

Ingredients
For the cake...
- 1 ½ cups (145g) almond flour
- ½ cup (65g) coconut flour
- 3 tablespoons stevia
- 2 tablespoons poppy seeds
- 2 teaspoons baking powder
- ½ teaspoon xanthan gum
- ½ cup (115g) butter, melted
- ½ cup (125ml) whipping cream
- Juice & zest from 2 lemons
- 2 large free-range eggs

For the topping...
- 3 tablespoons stevia
- ½ cup (120ml) boiling water
- 2 tablespoons butter, melted
- 2 tablespoons lemon juice

Method
1. Firstly take a few moments to line your slow cooker with aluminum foil and set to one side.
2. Now grab a bowl, add the almond flour, coconut flour, poppy seeds, stevia, baking powder and xanthan gum. Mix well until combined.
3. In a separate bowl, whisk the eggs with the butter, whipping cream, lemon juice and zest until lovely and light.
4. Then pour the dry mix into the wet mix, stir well to combine and pour into your slow cooker pan. Set to one side whilst we make the topping.
5. Grab another bowl and combine all the topping ingredients, stir well to combine and then pour over the cake batter waiting in your crock pot.
6. Cover with the lid and then cook on high for 2-3 hours until cooked through.
7. Serve and enjoy!

The Best Chocolate Cake You'll Taste All Year!

Quite a grand claim, don't you think? But as you're about to see, this chocolate cake really does deliver. Beautifully moist, achingly delicious and completely Keto-friendly, you just won't be able to resist eating a huge chunk. But don't worry- you'll still shift weight even if you eat it! Brilliant!

Serves: 10
Time: 2-3 hours

Ingredients
- 1 ½ cups almond flour
- ¾ cup stevia
- 2/3 cup unsweetened cocoa powder
- ¼ cup chocolate flavored protein powder
- 2 teaspoons baking powder
- ¼ teaspoon salt
- ½ cup unsalted butter, melted
- 4 large free-range eggs
- ¾ cup heavy cream
- 1 teaspoon vanilla extract

☐Method
1. First grease your slow cooker pan and set to one side.
2. The take a bowl and add the almond flour, stevia, cocoa powder, protein powder, baking powder and salt. Stir well to combine.
3. Next add the butter, eggs, cream and vanilla and give it a good stir until combined.
4. Pour the batter into your slow cooker pan and cook for 2 ½ to 3 hours on low. Keep checking until the cake is at your desired consistency then remove from the slow cooker pan and leave to cool.
5. Serve and enjoy!

Extras

Cajun Seasoning

Make your own Cajun seasoning for even better flavor and enjoyment.

Ingredients
- 2 1/2 tablespoons paprika
- 2 tablespoons salt
- 2 tablespoons garlic powder
- 1 tablespoon black pepper
- 1 tablespoon onion powder
- 1 tablespoon cayenne pepper
- 1 tablespoon dried oregano
- 1 tablespoon dried thyme

Method
1. Pour all the ingredients into a bowl, stir well and store in an airtight container until needed.
2. Serve and enjoy!

Avocado Cilantro Lime Sauce

Sure- this sauce doesn't require a slow cooker but it's perfect when served with chili verde so I thought I'd include it anyway.

Serves: 8
Takes: 2-3 minutes

Ingredients
- 1 avocado, pit removed and peeled
- 2 tablespoons cilantro, chopped
- Juice of ½ lime
- 2 teaspoons hot sauce
- 2 tablespoons sour cream

Method
1. Place all the ingredients into the blender, hit that button and whizz until perfectly creamy.
2. Serve and enjoy!

Zucchini Tortillas

Again, you won't be able to cook these in your slow cooker as they require an oven (sorry!), but they're the perfect Keto accompaniment for any meal you might choose to serve up, especially if it's Mexican-inspired so I decided to share the recipe with you anyway. Enjoy!

Serves: 2
Time: 15 mins

Ingredients
- 2 small zucchinis
- 2 cloves garlic, minced
- ½ teaspoon chili power
- Pinch salt and pepper, to taste
- 1 egg, beaten
- 1 teaspoon ground flax seed
- 1 tablespoons coconut flour

Method
1. Start by preheating your oven to 400F and lining a baking sheet with baking paper.
2. Place the zucchini and garlic into the food processer and blend until smooth.
3. Grab a cheese cloth or a clean tea towel and squeeze out as much liquid as you can. Pop into a large bowl and add the rest of the ingredients. Stir well until combined.
4. Take large spoons of this batter and pour onto the parchment paper, spreading to form large circles (but not too thin!)
5. Bake for 10-15 minutes then flip and bake again for a further 8-10 minutes.
6. Serve and enjoy!

NOTE: You can also fry these tortillas if preferred.

Final Words...

Whether you've been struggling with your weight since childhood, having a baby has really piled on the pounds or you're simply looking to up your endurance game and perform better as a human, I want you to know that **you can do this thing**.

You can shift the weight and return to your most awesome self. You can discover the untapped potential lying there inside you. You can make those lifestyle tweaks and watch the weight fall off, get stronger and healthier, grow in confidence and finally stand up tall and be proud of everything you are and everything you're capable of.

All it takes it that first step and you will show the world just what you're made of.

So don't just learn about Keto, nod your head in interest, bookmark the most interesting recipes and then just forget about this book. Actually take what you've learned and put it into action.

Life is too short to postpone until tomorrow. Start living right now. No excuses. No second chances- just grab life by the horns and do this thing!

Start making these Keto recipes, give the Ketogenic diet a chance, go and look up support groups near you and watch your life transform for the better. And don't forget- I'll be right beside you, cheering you on!

Before I go...

I almost forgot to say thanks for grabbing this book! I've had a wonderful time creating it and I hope you have an equally great time reading your way through it.

If you're enjoyed this book and you'd like to share your positive thoughts, please take a moment to leave me a review on Amazon. This small action will help me to keep sharing my Keto wisdom with the world and help people just like you to change their lives.

Again, thank you.

Appendix: Conversion Tables

As you might be aware, systems of measurement differ between the US, Canada, Australia and the UK. It can get pretty confusing if you're trying to follow a recipe using cups when you're not familiar with them, or trying to convert a temperature from Fahrenheit to Celsius or vice versa!

That's why you'll find both imperial and metric measurements in all recipes, along with temperature conversions.

But to make life a little easier for you and to help you investigate the world of amazing Ketogenic recipes even further, I've also put together these short conversion tables as an added bonus.

Oven Temperatures

Celsius	Fahrenheit
140°	285°
150°	300°
160°	320°
170°	338°
180°	356°
200°	392°
220°	425°
225°	437°

Liquid Volumes

mL	U.S.	fl oz
5	1 tsp	
15	1 tbsp	1/2
30	1/8 c	1
60	1/4 c	2
78	1/3 c	
118	1/2 c	4
158	2/3 c	
177	3/4 c	6
237	1 c	8
355	1 1/2 c	12
474	2 c	16
710	3 c	24
946	4 c	32

Dry Weights

grams	oz — lb
28	1
57	2
85	3
113	4oz — 1/4 lb
151	1/3 lb
227	8 oz. — 1/2 lb
302	2/3 lb
340	12 oz. — 3/4 lb
454	1 lb
907	2 lb

Made in the USA
Middletown, DE
29 November 2017